GW01444980

0

I dedicate this book to my partner Helen Renée.
She inspires me every day, in every way.

The △ISO90™ Course

The 90 Day/12 Week

Brutally Effective, Strength and Body Shaping Couse.

A Complete Course to Make You Strong

And Get You Into Shape FAST

Published by

MajorVision International

2017

△ISOfitness™

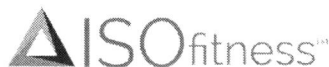

4

Contents

www.ISOfitness.us www.MajorVision.com www.ISOfitness.uk

Chapter1: Important General Safety and Health Guidelines

This section entitled, "Important General Safety and Health Guidelines," pertains to The ISOfitness™ Exercise System, and all books and publications about it, The ISO90™ Course, Fitness on the Move™, The 70 Second Difference™, The Bullworker Bible™, the Sixty Second Ass Workout™, The Bullworker 90™ Course, The Helen Renée™ Exercise System, or the Iso-Bow® System, recommendations, coaching, and advice, either written, verbal, in audio format, on video, written, or implied, from Brian Sterling-Vete and Helen Renée Wuorio, and the works thereof.

You should never begin any kind of sport, exercise system, or workout plan, including everything contained in The Bullworker 90™ Course, and in the beginning paragraph above, unless you have consulted and have the full approval of your medical doctor.

Your physician can properly assess your current health status, and your ability to perform the exercises in the book and/or course. This is particularly important if you have any known pre-existing health issues, you're pregnant, or if you believe that may have other serious health conditions.

It's essential that you must always have the absolute approval from your physician before starting. Please show all material in the above courses, books, video/audio, online material, and their content to your physician and get their approval before you start.

All exercises, suggestions, recommendations, instructions, exercise plans, dietary and eating recommendations, either given or implied, are intended only as a reference, and they are no substitute for a qualified professional personal coach who can help you to plan an exercise and diet program appropriate for your age and physical condition. Never overexert yourself when performing any exercise.

Stop exercising immediately and consult your doctor if you ever experience any pain, irregular heartbeat, shortness of breath, tightness in your chest/arms/fingers, faintness, nausea, or feelings of dizziness. Then consult your doctor, or call the EMS immediately.

The exercises, courses, plans, and dietary recommendations in The Bullworker90™ Course, and those mentioned in paragraph 1 of this section, are not intended for use by children. Keep all exercise equipment out of the reach of children.

Always inspect The Bullworker®, The Bow Extension®, the Iso-Bow®, and any/all exercise equipment before each use to ensure its proper operation, and to ensure that it is undamaged, and safe. Do not use it unless all parts are free from wear, and it is functioning properly. To avoid serious injury, care should always be taken using any/all exercise equipment, and in all items, people, books and courses, mentioned in paragraph 1 of this section.

Care should always be taken when getting into all exercise positions, on and off the floor, on and off chairs, on and off benches, on and off any other surface that might be used for exercise, including pieces of furniture, and in the use of The Bullworker®, The Bow Extension®, the Iso-Bow®.

The creators, writers, instructors, originators, and owners of The Bullworker90™ Course, The ISO90 Course™, and all publications on video, audio, and in print, together with the courses, and websites, owned, originated, and created by the copyright holders and the ISOfitness team, including all books, courses, and people mentioned in paragraph 1 of this section, accept no responsibility whatsoever for any injury, harm, damage, illness, or any negative health related condition which may occur as a direct, or indirect, result of following these courses, recommendation, or while performing any exercises.

For additional general information we also recommend that you check reputable accredited medical advice sites, such as the two listed below.

The National Health Service in the United Kingdom, online at: https://www.nhs.uk/Livewell/fitness/pages/physical-activity-guidelines-for-adults.aspx

In the USA, The Mayo Clinic online: http://www.mayoclinic.org/healthy-lifestyle/fitness/in-depth/exercise/art-20047414

Chapter 2: Introduction

ISO90™ is a comprehensive and complete step-by-step 90-day/12week body shaping, bodybuilding and functional strength building course based on the ISOfitness™ system of isometric exercises.

Since The ISO90™ Course engages your body's natural Adaptive Response™ mechanism, it makes it ideal for both beginners, advanced athletes, and even professional-level athletes. This is because no matter what level you're already at when you start, the harder and more intensely you work, the faster your body will respond.

The ISO90™ Course focusses the appliance of science in practical exercise and functional strength building, and in doing so, it makes the ISO90™ perhaps the fastest, and most efficient way to get into shape, build muscle and get strong which has ever been devised in a 90-day course.

The ISO90™ Course is also designed with time, ease of use, and flexibility in mind. Therefore, you can enjoy and benefit from a professional-level workout literally anywhere, and on almost any location. We've received positive testimonials, and useful feedback, from many people in different countries who were some of our early followers and enthusiasts of this system thanks to our "The 70 Second Difference™" book.

By the time this course is published, Helen Renée and I will have thoroughly tried and tested all the exercises in this course on numerous occasions. It will also have been tried and tested by athletes and enthusiasts of all levels including one World champion, and several serious amateur sports and fitness enthusiasts, as well as even people who haven't exercised in decades.

Furthermore, Helen and I have tried and tested the exercise routines in the ISO90™ course on our global travels, which helped us to keep our promise of it delivering professional standard workout sessions on almost any indoor or outdoor location. We've even tested it in both spacious and cramped conditions, and in some places where it would have otherwise been typically almost impossible to enjoy any other sort of professional gym level of workout.

We've even tested the ISO90™ workout routines while on several transatlantic flights, on a London-bound high-speed rail trip, as car passenger on a road trip, on board a ship crossing the Mediterranean, on the ramparts of the famous Urquhart Castle on the banks of Loch Ness in Scotland, during a break from fell walking around Eskdale and Wast Water in the English Lake District, on TV outside broadcasts for a famous US TV network, and even on the remote beaches and rock coves in Cornwall, England.

With the ISOfitness™ exercise system and The ISO90™ Course, the choice of where and when you exercise is always *your* choice, and it's never a choice imposed on you due to the traditional confines and restrictions of less efficient ways of exercising which require heavy and bulky equipment. This is true "Fitness on the Move."

It's About Time...

Lack of time is the traditional enemy of strength, fitness and body building, and to a degree we've all been conditioned over the years to subconsciously believe that a workout session will take between 30 and 60 minutes to perform. Indeed, lack of time is widely recognised as being the number one reason why people either don't exercise, or why they stop exercising.

Even the most dedicated exercise enthusiast who has relatively easy access to traditional exercise equipment, will sooner or later be forced to skip workouts due to lack of time. The inevitable time-crunches of life, family, and work are something that we all face, and with seemingly increasing regularity when the demands of work are particularly intense.

This is hardly surprising, especially when one considers how long it takes to attend a traditional gym or fitness club to maintain a regular workout schedule. Being a member of a gym can be incredibly time consuming. In just one week, someone who exercises regularly, 3 evenings each week, can easily spend the equivalent of a full working day doing that. Even if the average workout or exercise class can be completed in 60 minutes, the travel time there and back, traffic delays, parking hassles, changing and shower room time, searching for a vacant locker, and waiting for equipment at peak times etc. can make a single gym visit a 3-hour ordeal.

Even traditional home exercise systems still require a significant time-commitment for them to be effective, and deliver the desired results. Even "convenient" traditional home gym systems will still usually require between 20 and 60 minutes of exercise time to complete a workout. Since The ISO90™ Course is based on the proven science of maximum efficiency ISOfitness™ exercises, it is almost impossible *not* to be able find the time you need to exercise, even on your busiest day.

Even an unfit beginner, can complete a balanced total-body workout routine in as little as 10 or 12 minutes, and with most of the 10 to 12-minute time-period being needed to rest and recover their breath between the exercises! A more advanced athlete can almost certainly perform a specialised, and extremely high intensity total-body workout routine in a similar time-period, or less.

If you suddenly find that your daily travel or business schedule doesn't allow you the luxury of even finding 10 to 12 minutes to complete the scheduled workout in The ISO90™ Course, then you can always revert to the basic routine found in our foundation of 7 basic exercises that work all the major muscle groups of the body as described in "The 70 Second Difference™" book. This will enable you to maintain the gains you've already made. Can anyone honestly say that they can't find just 70 seconds of spare time to exercise, even of the busiest day imaginable? The fact is that lack of time to exercise is no longer a viable excuse!

Helen Renée and I are proud to have devised The ISO90™ Course together, and we sincerely hope that you enjoy it. We already know that if you perform it faithfully and properly, that you'll make excellent gains in your levels of functional strength, fitness, as well as great improvements in the overall size and shape of your body.

What is ISOfitness™?

The ISOfitness™ exercise system is the name we use to cover all exercises we write about, and teach. The core of the ISOfitness™ exercise system is based solidly on the original, proven isometric science. However, the ISOfitness™ system is much more than that alone. It incorporates the new, advanced isometric exercise discoveries and techniques including, Dynamic Flexation™, Super-Slow Isotonic Flexation™, and the newly proven science of USB-UHT™ (Ultra Short Burst – Ultra High Intensity) exercises. The ISOFitness™ exercise system also includes our own resultant hybrid TRISOmetric™ exercise system.

The 70 Second Difference™ Book and The ISO90™ Course

"The 70 Second Difference™" book covers all aspects of the ISOfitness™ exercise system, including the science and practical application of all major forms of isometric exercises, the science of strength, muscle growth, weight-loss, nutrition, and other important things related to fitness, strength training, bodybuilding, and body shaping. It also contains a comprehensive 7 exercise workout routine that will exercise all the main muscles of the body in only 70 seconds of consecutive exercise time. There is even a choice of workout for beginner, intermediary, and advanced athlete.

"The 70 Second Difference™" book is designed to be the foundation base-reference guide which will support all the courses we produce, including this ISO90™ course. In taking this approach, it means that we won't be repeating ourselves, or at least when we do it will be kept to a minimum, and only because we believe that we need to reinforce some extremely important point/s.

16

ISOfitness™ Online - Your Audio-Video Exercise Library

One of our primary objective with the www.ISOfitness.us and www.ISOfitness.uk websites is to create the most comprehensive reference library available anywhere. One containing printed material, stills pictures, and online audio-video resources which cover all aspects of scientific, functional isometric exercise. In the autumn of 2017, this will also include Bullworker® exercises.

We also intend to provide the similar resources covering all other major types of exercise including: resistance training with weights, machines, and other devices, sports-specific exercises and drills covering speed, quickness, agility, and power, together with a comprehensive range of martial arts related drills for Muay Thai, Western Boxing and other martial arts systems.

The majority of these have already been videoed and edited into both short clip form, and into several complete reference videos of up to an hour in length. These individual video clips and the complete edited course combination are designed to support every part of the ISOfitness™ exercise concept. Being able to view individual exercise clips on video makes it much easier to either examine specific exercises and techniques in much greater detail. They also serve as an extremely useful resource of different exercises for each body part to keep your daily workout routines fun, interesting and exciting.

In addition to this, we're also including immediately as a bonus to all ISOfitness™ website members, access to the 'Master Series' of sports-specific, fitness, martial arts, MMA, Boxing, athletics, and strength training related

17

videos. These videos provide comprehensive instruction on the development of attributes such as speed, agility, power, strength, core stability, martial arts/MMA/boxing bag work, speed ball, and focus mitt training, together with a resource library for exer-ball, bands/tubes, dumbbell training, and medicine ball drills.

The online video resource library of ISOfitness™ exercises already consists of 134 different isometric Iso-Bow® exercises at the time of writing this. With the current video production schedule, this resource library is set to grow to somewhere in the region of 350+ different exercise clips in total. This doesn't include the several hundred instructional clips of other types of exercise we have already to upload and release. Keep checking the members-side of the ISOfitness websites to see the latest video uploads as we grow the resource.

We're also very close to completing our ALL-NEW TRISOmetric™ exercise course book, complete with accompanying online videos. This is a very advanced 12-week, 90-day strength training and body building course. It's aimed specifically at advanced athletes and sports enthusiasts to take their training to the next level. It focusses very specifically on bodybuilding and body shaping using a highly advanced triple combination of scientifically proven exercise concepts. We've used our 40+ years of experience in the science of isometrics and bodybuilding to combine these elements in a complete, practical step-by-step 90-day, 12-week course. Advanced athletes can also any one, or any combination of several TRISOmetric™ exercises as part of their regular workout routine.

Chapter 3 – The 'How To' Part

Don't Forget the Science!

There are three basic types of resistance training. One type is isometric, which are exercises performed without any measurable movement of the limb being involved. The second type is isotonic exercise, which is all about movement. The third is isokinetic exercise, which is also about movement, however, with certain modifications to standard isotonic exercise applying to speed, velocity and force. Isokinetic exercises are not as commonly practiced as regular isotonic exercises.

An exercise is isotonic when the tension remains the same, whilst the length of the muscle changes, such as when lifting and lowering a weight. There are two parts to an isotonic contraction, these are: concentric (lifting) and eccentric (lowering). In a concentric contraction, the muscle tension rises to meet the resistance, then remains the same as the muscle shortens. In the eccentric, the muscle lengthens due to the resistance being greater than the force the muscle is producing.

Isokinetic and isotonic contractions appear to be the same, however, they are technically very different. During exercise, an isotonic contraction will keep force at a constant, while velocity changes. An isokinetic contraction will keep velocity at a constant, while the force changes. In other words, no matter how much effort is applied the velocity remains fixed, however, the resistance experienced by the muscles through the limb's range of motion will change. Isokinetic exercises can be performed very effectively with an Iso-Bow®.

All three are excellent at building strength, and muscle size, as well as providing many other physical and health-related benefits. However, science has proven that one properly performed isometric exercise at only 2/3rds of an individual's overall maximum can deliver either similar, or often better results, than the equivalent of up to 3 sets of 10 weight training repetitions. This is because, when performed properly, and at the correct level of intensity, isometric exercise engages many more muscle fibres than can be achieved with regular weight training.

Comparison studies were carried out at the world-famous Max Plank institute in Dortmund, Germany, over a 5-year period. The results of these experiments were published in the ground-breaking book: 'The Physiology of Strength,' by Dr. Theodor Hettinger. They performed over 5,500 experiments on volunteers from all walks of life, from all age groups, on both sexes, and at every level of strength and fitness. The results were revolutionary, because they revealed the superiority of isometric exercise in building both strength and muscle much faster, and comparatively easier, than isotonic exercise could. They also revealed something equally remarkable. This was that after performing only a single 7-second training stimulus (exercise) per day, the muscle being exercised was no longer responsive to further gains. The scientific data about this can be referenced on pages 28 to 31 of Dr. Theodor Hettinger's book, "The Physiology of Strength."

Therefore, we don't typically recommend performing more than one isometric exercise in each position for each muscle group. The exception to this rule would be if a more advanced athlete wanted to develop a more constant strength-curve throughout the practical operational motion of a limb. This is because typically, the maximum strength gains during an isometric exercise are at the point which the isometric hold takes place, with additional benefits being gained in a strength-curve of as much as +20% and -20% of that initial point. Therefore, even an advanced athlete would probably only need to perform the isometric exercise at 2, or possibly 3 points, along the entire range of motion of the limb. Another exception, would if an advanced or professional level athlete was employing a TRISOmetric™ exercises technique.

Another compelling research study revealed that the levels of muscle activation during repetitions of maximal weight training were between 89.7%, during the concentric contraction, or the lifting a weight, and 88.3% during the eccentric contraction, or the lowering of a weight. For practical purposes, about 89%. Scientific measurement also showed that during the lifting, or concentric, part of the exercise, the maximum intramuscular tension only lasted for between 0.25 and 0.5 seconds. Again, for practical purposes, about 1/3rd of a second. This is because traditional isotonic resistance exercises naturally involve movement, therefore, they also have aspects of velocity and acceleration to consider. Furthermore, "force" is only produced for a split second, to produce a maximal contraction of the muscle fibres.

However, the same research also clearly proved that the level of muscle activation during isometric exercise was as high as 95.2%, and that it lasted for the entire 7 to 10 second period of each exercise. In addition to this, the muscle activation also lasted for 7 to 10 second period of the isometric exercise, which is a huge increase over the $1/3^{rd}$ of second muscular activation achieved during a single repetition of weight training. In practical terms, this means that if you're prepared to perform one daily isometric exercise for just 7 seconds, and at only $2/3^{rd}$'s of your maximum effort, then it's possible to increase your strength by an average of up to 5% per week. If you can expect strength gains of an average of 5% per week in exchange for the expenditure of only $2/3^{rd}$'s of your maximum effort, it's an excellent result!

As with all ISOfitness™ advanced isometric exercises, performing Iso-Bow® exercises will engage your body's natural Adaptive Response™ mechanism. Therefore, if you always aim to perform the highest quality exercise, and at the highest level of intensity, you'll gain the maximum benefits possible in the shortest possible time. You can expect to become stronger, and fitter after each workout session. This then means that for your next exercise session you will be a little stronger and fitter than you were for your previous session, which in turn means that you're able to put even more effort and intensity into your new exercise session, than you did into the previous one. The cycle will then continue until you reach a physical plateau which is determined by your natural physical characteristics, capabilities, your age, and sex.

In respect of pure bodybuilding, even though isometric exercise is excellent at increasing muscle fibre density, size, and strength, pure bodybuilding requires an additional approach to deliver the maximum desired results. In pure bodybuilding, the quest isn't merely for strength, instead, it's all about muscle size, shape and

23

aesthetics. Strength athletes would typically focus their training more on the prime mover muscles needed for strength related events. Bodybuilders will more widely spread the focus of their training to cover more of the muscle groups they want to develop. Isometric exercise will achieve both goals. However, the addition of the controlled pumping action of Dynamic Flexation™ will help to maximise both goals more efficiently.

Workout Intensity Concepts

"Intensity" is always going to be a relative term, and it's often completely misunderstood when it's used in relation to exercise. Basically, when it comes to exercising your muscles, intensity is the % of your ability to move a resistance. Technically, an individual's highest possible level of intensity is when they reach a point of momentary failure after exerting themselves completely. However, in practical terms the important questions we need to try and find answers to are: "How hard is hard?" and "How intense is intense?" To some degree, both are both very subjective things. Taking two people of roughly equal fitness, something that is intense to one person might be considered comparatively easy to the other.

"Hard" is also a relative term, and even 50lbs of resistance is impossibly hard if your strength is only at the level required to lift 49lbs. However, if you're able to lift a 100lbs as a maximum, then lifting 50lbs is going to be comparatively easy. Often, the only factors differentiating between people and the intensity level exerted, are going to be mental toughness, determination, and perception.

24

The human brain has a built-in mechanism which helps to protect the body and prevent it from performing physical activity to such a level that could cause serious damage, or even death. This is the mechanism that makes your brain tell you to stop exercising when it begins to get tough, and the feeling of wanting to stop exercising, only increases as you continue to push yourself harder to do more. This is all despite the biological fact that you're physically capable of doing much more than is being suggested by the messages you're receiving from yourself.

Over time, the brain of people who exercise regularly, and especially to a high level of intensity, will naturally adjust and reposition this built-in safety margin. In practical terms, this means that the brain of an experienced high-level athlete doesn't "tell" them to stop an exercise until the level of intensity is much higher than it would be for a beginner. Therefore, when it comes to exercise, how is it possible to subjectively quantify, and then impart appropriate levels of recommended intensity? This problem is made even more challenging when one considers the fact that accurately translating and subjectively assessing various levels of intensity will, to some degree, always be subjective to every individual.

If you really do train as hard as it's humanly possible to train, with near 100% maximum intensity, which involves super-strict form, training to complete failure, and beyond, then you simply can't train for a long period of time. It's just physiologically impossible. The physics and biology are very simple in this respect. The intensity of your workout is directly proportional to the length of time that you're physically able to perform your workout. The harder and more intensely you exercise, then the shorter time that you'll be physically able perform the exercise. Make no mistake, performing a 7 second isometric exercise while exerting close to your personal 100% maximum physical capacity is completely and utterly exhausting, even for a professional athlete. In practical terms, what does all of this mean when it comes to accurately communicating various levels of exercise intensity, especially when there's no professional coach, or elaborate and expensive measuring equipment at hand?

The first, and most obvious thing to remember, is that research clearly shows that almost everyone will stop exercising long before they're in any danger of becoming seriously fatigued. In other words, most people will *"think"* they're achieving a much higher level of intensity than they would do if they were only a little more mentally resilient. This doesn't mean that people should suddenly begin pushing themselves beyond their physical limits, which would be a stupid thing to do. However, it does mean that most people who enjoy a higher than average level of mental resilience and determination, as well as being in physically good condition, can push themselves much harder than they might think. Naturally, if anyone ever feels "genuine" strain, or fatigue to the point of becoming injured, then they should stop exercising immediately.

Even without the aid of a professional coach to monitor, encourage you and measure your intensity and progress with specialist equipment, the tips we've outlined in this section will help you to get the most out every workout. It's also worth remembering that if you cheat, then the only person who really loses every time is "YOU."

Dynamic Flexation™

We'll recap and briefly summarise the Dynamic Flexation™ technique as laid out in "The 70 Second Difference™" book. Even for a beginner, we would always recommend that to some degree everyone employs a form of Dynamic Flexation™. This will help to ensure that all muscles, tendons, ligaments, joints, and spine become naturally and properly engaged in the correct isometric exercise position, which will usually be helped by taking a correct hand grip, fist clench, or foot position.

This means that you should always ensure that you perform each exercise in the correct biomechanical position to gain maximum benefit from each exercise. When you assume the correct position, to begin with you should apply almost no tension whatsoever. Instead, you should "feel" your way into ensuring that you're in the correct position *before* beginning to apply tension to the exercise. Once you're in the correct position, perhaps the worst thing to do would be to suddenly apply maximum tension, and at the same time hold your breath. This is completely wrong. Instead, remember to always breathe naturally as you gradually engage your muscles into the exercise.

Our personal preference is to apply the tension gradually through Dynamic Flexation™, over a period of up to 3 or even 4 seconds. This is before beginning to count the required 7-second exercise hold of the isometric contraction. During the exercise, be sure to breathe naturally and deeply. We prefer using each full breath in and out as a method of counting more accurately the number of seconds each exercise is performed, with one breath in and out representing one second. Similarly, at the

27

end of an exercise we don't recommend that it be ended abruptly. Instead, we prefer to reverse the Dynamic Flexation™ technique, and to gradually relax and slightly move each muscle and joint as you do so.

Dynamic Flexation™ is a concept which embraces the broader principles of motor unit recruitment, and "Henneman's Size Principle," to increase the contractile strength of a muscle. Elwood Henneman's principle stated that, under load, the motor units in a muscle are engaged according to their magnitude of force output, from the smallest to the largest, and in task-appropriate order. This means that the slow-twitch, low-force, fatigue-resistant muscle fibres are activated before any fast-twitch, high-force muscle fibres are engaged which are less fatigue-resistant. Since the body works in this way, it enables precise, finely controlled force to be delivered at all levels of output. In practical terms, this also means that when exercising, or when performing tasks in daily life, the fatigue which is experienced as a result will be always be minimised, and proportional to the sequential engagement of the most appropriate muscle fibres.

Cardio, ISOfitness™, and Rest Time Between Exercises

Early in The ISO90™ Course you'll find that we include some "introductory" and "optional" cardio exercise recommendations in addition to the isometric exercises in the routine. You'll also note that shortly afterwards there are no further recommendations for the inclusion of cardio exercise with the later sections of the course. This is because if you keep the rest time between exercises brief enough, then the ISO90™ workout routine itself will give

28

you an excellent cardiovascular workout, and this is what we recommend that you ultimately aim for.

If you're already very fit, then we'd recommend that instead of performing the optional cardio routine, and you simply put more effort and intensity into each ISO90™ isometric exercise. At the same time, aim to keep the rest time between those exercises as brief as possible. This approach will help you work towards being able to perform each exercise so that it has an Ultra-High Intensity Ultra-Short Burst™ effect, which will greatly improve your overall fitness level, and boost your Base Metabolic Rate or BMR. However, if you're not already fit, then to begin with you may wish to simply allow each isometric exercise to deliver all the cardio you need as you gradually build up your levels of fitness and endurance. Eventually, you'll soon increase your level of fitness to a point where you can begin to significantly, and steadily, reduce the rest time between each exercise to a minimum point that works best for you.

Once you've learned how to fully engage the muscles during each exercise with sufficient intensity, and at the same time you've learned how to breathe fully, deeply, and naturally throughout each exercise, while at the same time keeping the rest time between exercises to a minimum, then this combination will have an excellent and beneficial cardiovascular effect.

Ultra-High Intensity, Ultra-Short Burst™

Short bursts of high intensity exercise are extremely effective at breaking down the body's stored reserves of glucose in the muscles, which is called glycogen. When these reserves of glycogen are rapidly depleted due to the

29

high intensity bursts of exercise, it creates room for the glucose in your blood to replace it and be stored instead. In short, it removes some of the sugar circulating in your bloodstream, which in turn has both overall health and weight loss benefits.

Research carried out by Professor Jamie Timmons of Nottingham University in England conducted a four-year detailed scientific study with over 1000 test subjects about the efficacy of Ultra-High Intensity Ultra-Short Burst™ exercise in comparison with other types of exercise. Unsurprisingly, they found that the key to gaining the greatest benefits from exercise were based in extremely short high intensity exercise sessions, and not in lengthy, prolonged workouts.

However, their research also concluded something quite remarkable which is that as little as 3 minutes per week of ultra-high intensity exercise, performed in extremely short bursts of only 10 seconds each, is all that's needed to significantly boost a person's Base Metabolic Rate (BMR), dramatically improve cardiovascular efficiency, improve their overall health, and get them into great shape too.

This 10 second "magic" number for a basic Ultra-High Intensity Ultra-Short Burst™ exercise routine is a perfect length of exercise time. This is because it coincides perfectly with the 7 seconds of time needed to perform a practical high intensity isometric exercise, together with the few extra seconds of exercise which are always needed to properly engage, and then disengage the muscles and joints. This means that when performed at a very high level of intensity, isometric exercises have a similar effect to a basic Ultra-High Intensity Ultra-Short Burst™ exercise routine. Beyond this Ultra-High Intensity Ultra-Short Burst™ advanced isomeric exercise effect, advanced and professional athletes can then factor-in the amount of rest time taken between exercises.

According to the highly acclaimed and pioneering sports scientist, Arthur Jones, the man who invented the famous Nautilus system, muscle recovery has a half-life which occurs every 3 seconds after an exercise has been stopped. This means that in as little as 9 seconds of rest time you're ready to begin your next exercise. Naturally, 9 seconds is an extremely brief period, and after performing an extremely high intensity exercise your heart and lungs will be working exceptionally hard.

Therefore, aiming for a consistent 9 second rest time target between each exercise is going to be incredibly challenging, and it's something which is only possible for people who are already exceptionally fit, advanced, semi-pro, and professional athletes. In practical terms though, especially when beginning exercises for the first time, most people will take a much longer rest period between exercises, especially if they're performed at an average of approximately 2/3rds of someone's personal maximum capacity.

We'd suggest that you don't rush any of this, and that only as you gradually improve your levels of fitness, then you can also aim to gradually reduce the amount of rest time taken between exercises. We'd always recommend that you always practice maximum caution in all things, especially when it comes to pushing yourself to new, higher limits in your workout routine.

Always do this with safety in mind, take your age and physical ability into consideration, and never to push yourself beyond your personal safe limits. This would be the safest, and most efficient way to work towards the goal of performing each exercise in The ISO90™ Course as an Ultra-High Intensity Ultra-Short Burst™ exercise, followed by only a maximum of 9 to 10 seconds of rest time between each exercise. At this point you'll be giving yourself one of the most effective cardiovascular workouts possible, while you'll also be performing the most efficient strength and muscle building exercises possible. Which is a double-win all around!

Therefore, if you want to perform any additional cardio or other sports-related exercises, that would be fine. We'd always highly recommend an overall active lifestyle, and especially participation in sport of all kinds, especially potentially practical ones like the martial arts. The only recommendation we'd make is that you do them after, and separately to the exercises and routines in The ISO90™ Course. Also, don't forget to compensate and accommodate for any additional exercise you take and energy expenditure in your overall rest, recovery, and nutritional plan.

Strength, Stamina, Endurance, and Resilience

It is important to understand the difference between strength, stamina and endurance, because once understood, you'll then be able to devise the most suitable workout routines according to your body type.

Muscular strength is possibly best understood as being a muscle's capacity to exert force against resistance, or weight. This is comparatively easy to measure because your ability to lift a given amount of weight for a single repetition is a good measure of your strength.

Stamina is the length of time at which a muscle, or group of muscles, can perform at or near your maximum capacity. For example, the number of squats you can perform with a given weight which is 90% of your maximum would be a measure of your stamina, or the distance which you can carry a similar heavy object such as an anvil.

Endurance is all about time, and your ability to perform a certain muscular action for a prolonged period regardless of the capacity at which you're working.

Resilience is all about your ability to recover from whatever stresses and demands are placed upon your muscles. However, resilience is mostly all about your state of mind, your mental toughness and ability to endure, perform and deliver under pressure, and to recover quickly emotionally.

The muscular composition of your body will always determine how well you will perform at certain sports. The amount of slow twitch muscle fibres you possess will determine how well you perform at endurance related events, and both type A and type B fast twitch muscle fibres are all about explosive power and your ability to maintain it.

In simple terms, if you possess mostly slow twitch fibres, then you're naturally be better suited to endurance sports. Alternatively, if you possess mostly fast twitch muscle fibres, then you're a natural weight lifter. It's important to note, that no matter what your natural predisposition might be in this respect, with the correct training regimen, it is still possible to significantly increase your abilities in your naturally weaker opposing areas of speciality.

Rest and Recovery

For those who have already read about this subject in "The 70 Second Difference™" book, they will know that rest and recovery after intense exercise is essential. This is because your body, and immune system, must be given sufficient time to recuperate properly.

In addition to this, if it's your intention to significantly increase your muscle size and strength, then it's always worth remembering that your muscles don't grow during your workout. The workout phase is the stimulus, and the real growth process begins after your workout is over, during the recovery period.

Exercising too often will prevent complete recovery from taking place, and it will eventually deplete your muscle tissue, and have the completely opposite effect to what you wish to achieve. When calculating your ideal recovery period many things must be taking into consideration including: your age, your current health and fitness level, the quantity of exercise taken, and most importantly the intensity of the exercise which has been performed.

Some people will need a recovery period of between 24 and 48 hours, and for others the recovery period may be as brief as between 12 and 24 hours. However, as a rule, the recovery period will incrementally increase as the intensity of the exercises increases towards an individual's 100% potential maximum capacity.

Sports scientist J. Atha's research revealed something remarkable. This was that when performing isometric contraction exercises at 2/3rd's of an individual's maximum capacity, the average person could safely perform an exercise like this daily, without overtraining.

This means that the isometric exercises in The ISO90™ Course can be safely performed daily, by almost anyone, of almost any age, and in almost any physical condition as a means of strength development, body shaping, and even for bodybuilding. However, you'll notice in The ISO90™ Course that we recommend several variations in workout frequency and recovery periods. For some workouts which are performed at specific recommended levels of intensity, there may be no recovery time, and the exercise next session will be performed the next day. For other workouts, especially when starting The ISO90™ Course, and then also later in the course following a particularly intense workout period, we will recommend a rest day between workouts due to the higher demands being placed upon the Central Nervous System (CNS).

There are several other factors which affect post-exercise recovery. These include a balanced and properly executed stretching routine, and getting enough quality sleep. While you sleep, your body releases certain hormones which help you to repair and rebuild damaged tissue, and which will directly help your muscles to grow.

Post exercise high quality nutrition will help your body to repair itself faster, decrease your recovery time, and will help to generally maximise the benefits gained from the exercise.

Studies indicate that there is a 30 to 60-minute time-window after exercise when you need to eat, and after which, your body begins to draw upon itself to repair and recover from your exercise session. Drinking enough water is also one of the most important factors in your recovery, as well as for your overall health, because your muscles are mostly composed of water.

Biceps, Supination, and Strong Arms

When most people think about the biceps muscles, they only think about flexing the biceps and elbow joint to create a classic bodybuilder biceps pose. However, there is a great deal more to the biceps muscles than this.

While flexing the arm in the way I've just described might be a primary function, another equally primary function is the action of twisting the forearm and hand, otherwise known as supination.

Supination starts with the hand in a neutral position, roughly parallel to the side of your upper thigh, and twisting it as it is being raised until your

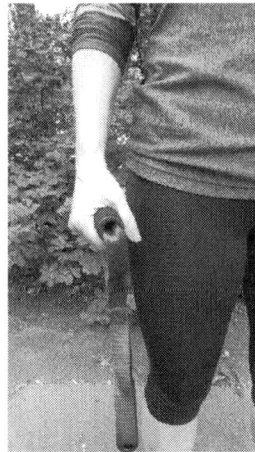

Neutral Position Front

palm is facing upwards at the top of the movement when the biceps are fully flexed.

The brachialis muscle is the primary mover of elbow flexion, and not the biceps brachii as most people think. This is because, even though the biceps brachii "show" muscle is seen flexed during a classic biceps pose, it is the brachialis which underlies it that generates about 50% more power than the biceps brachii. Therefore,

Mid Supination Side View

supination is not only important to elbow rotation, but to overall upper arm strength. Therefore, to gain maximum benefit and strength when exercising your overall front upper arm, all component muscles and their actions must be taken into consideration.

The problem with isometric exercise in this respect, when by pitting only limb against limb or static

Neutral Position Side View

immovable objects such as a wall, door or chair, doesn't naturally allow the brachialis muscle to be exercised effectively.

Mid Supination Front View

The Iso-Bow®, and the Bow Extension kit, offer an effective solution to this problem. These simple, yet highly effective devices allow a user to perform a wide range of exercises, either as a stand-alone device, or in combination with other devices such as the Bullworker® and/or Steel Bow®. More importantly, they enable effective

Full Supination Side View

isometric, and isotonic exercises to be performed in biomechanically correct ways.

Since the Iso-Bow® can be used to perform a wide range of barbell and dumbbell-like exercises either isometrically, or isotonically, this makes supination with the Iso-Bow® very easy. This makes it possible, and easy, to perform an isometric hold in both the neutral hand position, the semi-supinated hand position, and the fully supinated hand position. Naturally, the same rules of exercise speed of motion, breathing, and correct biomechanical positioning apply to all concentric, and eccentric actions. In respect of executing a biceps curl exercise in the best style possible, complete with supination, here are a few tips:

Full Supination Front View

⚠ As a rule, when performing a biceps curl, never allow your elbows to move forward, or kick-out to the side.

⚠ As with all curling exercises, never allow your wrist to bend backwards to fall out of alignment with the forearm, because in this position, you're between 3 and 4 times weaker than if you hand and wrist was locked in correct biomechanical alignment.

⚠ In the starting position of any biceps exercise, always begin by firstly flex the triceps a little to ensure that you've fully lengthened the biceps, which will help to maximise the range of motion.

⚠ You can always adjust your gripping position on a hand grip to create and off-centre position, because this will force your biceps to work even harder through supination.

Finally, I believe that it's important to remember that contrary to common belief, the strength-benefit of an isometric hold can be as high as +/- 20% of the position of the exercise.

Therefore, even by performing an exercise in only 1 position, it will still deliver a great deal of benefit in terms of muscle growth and in an overall increase in strength.

Supersets

A superset is when one performs two, or more, different physical exercises performed back-to-back, without a period of rest between them. The exercises typically target either the same, or opposing muscle groups. The only "rest" that is allowed during a superset is the amount of time to change between exercises, which should always be kept to a minimum anyway.

Supersets are ideal to use with opposing body parts, such as chest and back, or biceps and triceps. This is because the non-working muscles are not only rested and relaxed while their antagonists are exercised.

Supersets place an increased emphasis on the cardiovascular system, which helps to increase overall fitness levels while burning more calories and fat as a result. You'll be performing ISOfitness™ supersets in weeks 8 and 9 of The ISO90™ Course.

The Iso-Bow®

A common question we're asked is: "is it necessary to use the Iso-Bow® to perform an effective isometric or self-resisted workout?"
This is a very good question.

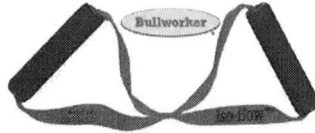

No, it's not necessary to use an Iso-Bow®, but we believe that it is better if you do, and there are several reasons why.

Firstly, it's all about the science and safety of biomechanics. A stable line of biomechanical progression all begins with a correctly positioned grip, a firm grip, and the progression in continuing that stability through correctly aligned joints and limbs while you perform the exercise.

The same is true in isometric exercise, because it all begins with a stable line of biomechanical progression starting with either a properly clenched hand or fist, and continuing that stability through correctly aligned joints and limbs to perform the isometric hold.

This is just one reason why we fully recommend and endorse the Iso-Bow®, because it makes this whole process much easier. It has a well-designed and comfortable non-slip hand grip, which allows you to execute a firm, stable hand grip position to begin creating a stable line of biomechanical progression.

The Iso-Bow® is a product we fully endorse and highly recommend. It's inexpensive, high quality, and it works exceptionally well. An amazing Iso-Bow® costs "pennies" in comparison to other exercise devices, and even a pair of them can easily fit into your pocket, they never need adjusting, they can deliver a total-body workout at the perfect level of intensity for either a complete unfit beginner, or an advanced athlete!

If you've already read "The 70 Second Difference™" Book, then you'll also know that we're not even endorsing our own product. We're simply endorsing a product which we believe will be the best investment you'll ever make if you want to get fit, strong, and in the best shape of your life. The company that makes the Iso-Bow® is Hughes Marketing LLC, and they also

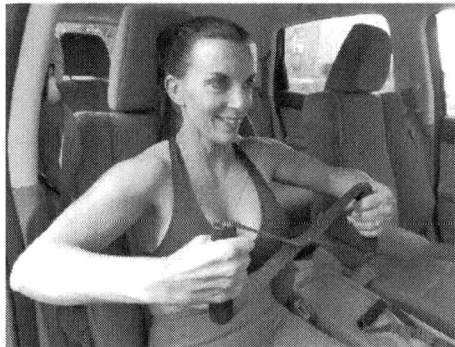

produce a small range of other high equally exercise products, which all deliver excellent results at a fair price.

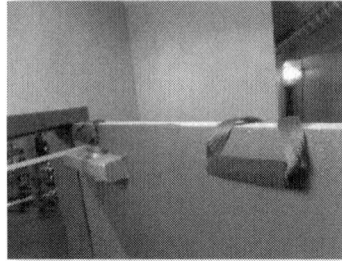

The Iso-Bow® is versatile too, and it can be used with equal effectiveness as both an isotonic, and an isometric exercise device. It allows the user to perform

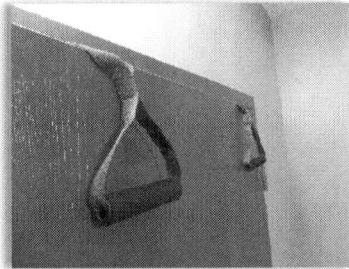

highly-effective self-resisted isotonic exercises for almost every muscle group.

A pair of Iso-Bows® can even be used as a great doorway pull-up device, which can even fold up and slip right into your pocket when you're done. Try doing that with a regular, clumsy steel doorway pull-up bar!

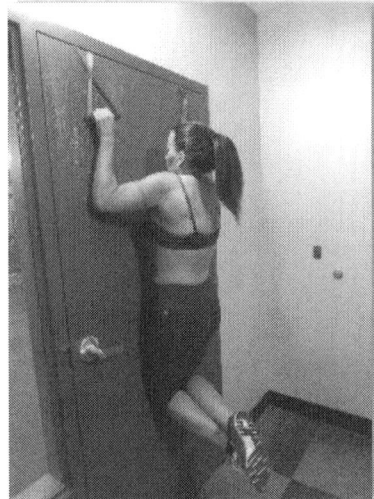

The Iso-Bow® is naturally a first-class isometric exercise device, and it allows a very wide range of exercises to be performed that work almost every muscle group of the body. It also allows the effective execution of more advanced techniques to be performed within the ISOfitness™ system.

Since the Iso-Bow® is so inexpensive, well designed, well-constructed, and extremely useful in ways we haven't even begun to describe here in this book, it's not so much a recommendation for you to get a pair, rather an instruction for you to do so. We believe that you'll soon see why these inexpensive devices are what we believe to be the finest, most versatile, and most powerful of all exercise devices which have ever been invented!

That's a bold statement, but it's made from our 'heart,' and it's delivered with our most sincere belief in the product and how you will benefit from owning a pair, and in using them correctly. Don't forget, we don't make this product, we simply believe in it to that degree of commitment.

Securing The Iso-Bow® With Your Feet

When performing leg exercises such as squats and lunges, as well as lower back and glute exercises such as deadlift, it becomes necessary to

properly secure the Iso-Bow® using your feet.

There are several ways in which the Iso-Bow® can be secured using your feet, and your personal preference of how you do this will depend upon many factors such as your foot size, your choice of footwear, and ease of operation.

You can secure the Iso-Bow® with your foot inside one of the handles. You do this by adjusting the hand grip to one side, usually the outer side of the foot, and then place your feet inside the loop like a stirrup.

Another method is to place the Iso-Bow® flat on the floor and then stand on one side of the straps so that the handle of the same side sits flush to your inner foot. In this position, it will be your bodyweight combined with the handle pressing against the inner side of your foot which enables you pull safely and securely.

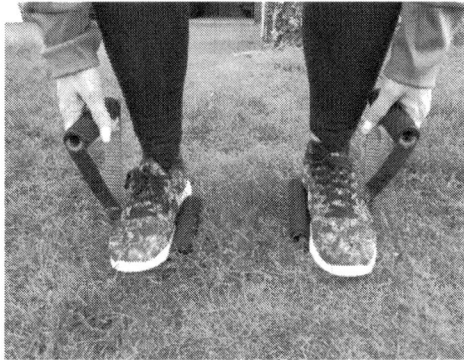

The final method is to simply place each foot through one end of an Iso-Bow®, stepping onto the foam hand grip as you do so. This method offers slightly less stability than the other two methods. However, if the foot can be pushed far enough

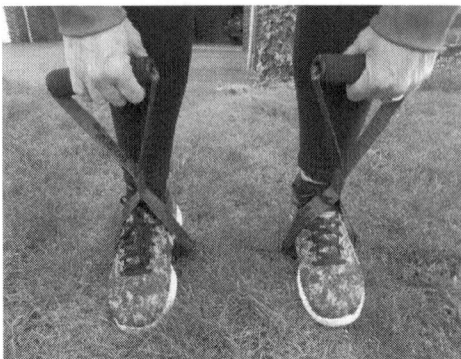

though the loop of the Iso-Bow® handle, then the handle will slightly raise the level of your heel making it easier for some people to squat or lunge.

Naturally, safety is always a top priority so whichever method you ultimately choose to use, you should always make sure that when securing the Iso-Bow® with your feet that there is never any chance of it slipping in any way while you exercise.

Shortening The Iso-Bow® - The Cradle

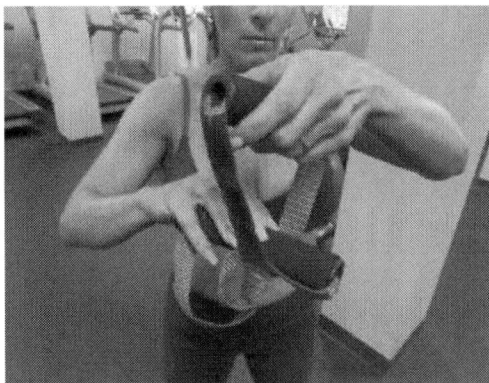

Generally, the Iso-Bow® is the ideal size for the most people to use with all exercises.

However, occasionally you may prefer to reduce its operational size by roughly half, by creating what we call an Iso-Bow® cradle.

To do this you place one of the handles inside the webbing loop of the other handle side of the device. The handle you've just placed inside the loop is then cradled by the webbing and can be gripped as normal. Your thumb, and fingers can then wrap around both the foam handle, and the webbing of the cradle-loop to help ensure an even firmer grip position is created.

This reduced size allows for an even greater operational range within the movement capability of each limb / joint to be created for certain exercises. These include: The Cross-Chest Press, The Upper Back Power Pull, and The Biceps and Triceps Cradle Press-Curl.

Before You Begin...

The first, and perhaps the most important thing to remember is: **NEVER HOLD YOUR BREATH AT ANY TIME, AND EACH DEEP BREATH WILL COUNT THE NUMBER OF SECONDS IN EACH EXERCISE**.

Always practice breathing naturally in and out before performing any exercise against resistance. When you have mastered the ability of being able to breathe in and out naturally while you perform each exercise, only then should you begin to apply increased resistance and intensity in the performance of the exercise.

Breathing in and out naturally during all isometric exercises will also to help you count the number of elapsed seconds much more accurately. This technique will help to ensure that you don't cheat by counting the seconds too quickly as you exercise. It's just natural for everyone to count a little too quickly when exercising. Don't feel bad about it, just use this technique to help prevent this happening, and to ensure that you get the very best results from your workout routines.

We recommend that you read the instructions about each workout routine and exercise carefully. You can also watch the associated videos on the ISOfitness™ website. We'd even recommend that you do this several times before starting each workout routine in the course.

You may well have already performed some, or even all the isometric exercises in The ISO90™ Course. However, you've almost certainly never done them exactly as we recommend them.

We're completely confident that the thoroughly tried, tested, and researched ISO90™ course will deliver all the results you want, and in the fastest way possible. We're also confident that you'll soon begin to see and feel results, in fact you'll probably feel the ISO90™ system working right from your very first workout.

Weight loss/fat loss will ONLY occur when The ISO90™ Course, or ANY other exercise plan, is used in conjunction with a calorie controlled diet.

This is obvious to most people, but there are always some who are clueless in this respect, or they claim to be. Even The 70 Second Difference™ book deliberately doesn't contain any diet plans, because everyone has different requirements in this respect. However, it contains all the science and nutrition information you need to make better food choices.

It's critically important to completely focus your mind on the exercise being performed, and in addition to this, to fully envision the muscle growing and getting stronger. This is because it's the neural pathways in the brain which conduct the stimuli needed to determine the intensely of the contractions within the muscle when it's being exercised.

With increased neural pathway capacity, the intensity of the muscular contraction which is produced also increases, and this makes the muscles grow larger and stronger as a result. So fully concentrate on the exercise you're performing, and envision in detail the results you want from them, and it really will help you to achieve them.

Always consult a professional coach to devise a detailed stretching routine, this will ensure that you're stretching the areas effectively rather than risk injury. Always ensure that a stable line of biomechanical progression is achieved before engaging in, and performing any exercise.

Warm-up Before Exercise - Stretch and Cool-Down After

Warming-up, stretching, and cooling down are three of the most overlooked, yet essential elements to exercise, and we cannot stress their importance strongly enough. During ANY form of physical exercise, including isometrics, if you apply too much intensity too soon, then you may inadvertently strain a muscle. Isometric exercise is particularly intense, and a single isometric exercise engages a great many more muscle fibres than even high intensity weight training, and isometrics engages the muscle fibres at a much higher level too.

Therefore, for safety's sake, we're adamant that you should always gradually and progressively engage your muscles into ANY isometric exercise, and according to what we call The ISOfitness Exercise Timeline™.

The main benefit to properly warming up for several minutes before a workout is injury prevention, because you'll increase your heart rate, circulation to your muscles, ligaments and tendons. It's important to remember that warming-up and stretching are two different concepts, and stretching isn't a good warm-up. This is because stretching will put the muscle in an un-contracted position, and weakening it. Stretching is always best performed after a workout has been completed, together with a proper cool-down.

In addition to properly warming-up, always perform a gentle "flex and stretch" of the muscles and joints which are about to be exercised. For example, squatting down fully to flex the thighs and loosen the knees is always a good idea before performing any leg exercises. Dynamic Flexation™ should always be used with every ISOfitness™ style isometric exercise. Here's a diagram which explains the workflow visually.

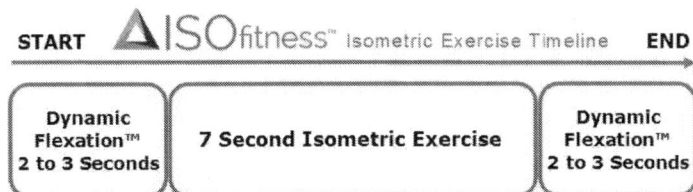

START △ISOfitness™ Isometric Exercise Timeline **END**

Dynamic Flexation™ 2 to 3 Seconds	7 Second Isometric Exercise	Dynamic Flexation™ 2 to 3 Seconds

ISOfitness™ style isometric exercises are deceptively powerful. Even when engaging in what may feel like only moderate intensity exercise, you're probably still engaging and contracting a great many more muscle fibres than you would in a similar isotonic exercise. Therefore, if you're in any doubt whatsoever, then always perform exercise with a little less intensity. In addition to a proper warm-up, the Dynamic Flexation™, performed in conjunction the isometric exercise, will help to ensure a greater blood supply to the muscles and surrounding tissue.

51

The ISO90™ Course, and ALL ISOfitness exercises and workout plans work equally well for men AND women. BOTH sexes can build great strength, solid muscle, body build, or simply get into great shape if they wish, each according to their natural potential.

Just because Helen Renée usually demonstrates the exercises in our printed products, stills pictures, and in the videos on the members-side of the ISOfitness™ website, it doesn't mean that the exercises and products are only for women. They're NOT!

The science, the exercises, the techniques, and the workout routines, all work equally well for both sexes at every level, from a complete beginner right up to a sports professional, bodybuilder, and strength athlete. Men who think this way, then get over any silly notion about this now! That's 'dinosaur' thinking!

Please read, review, and ensure that you've fully complied with all recommendations in the section entitled: 'The Obligatory BUT Highly Important General Safety and Health Recommendations,' and only start The ISO90™ Course with the full approval of your physician.

If you've done all of this, then you're all set to start your ISO90™ 12-week course to a build a totally new 'YOU!'

The ISO90™ Course Week 1

Week 1 Notes

△ Unless you're already fit and are someone who exercises regularly, then we'd recommend that for the first week of training you apply only approximately 50% of your maximum potential intensity to each exercise.

Perform only one 7 second isometric exercise contraction. *(Don't start counting until you've fully applied the desired level of intensity)*

△ Before you begin the full isometric contraction part of the exercise, take between 2 and 3 additional seconds to perform Dynamic Flexation™ to help you properly engage the muscles and joints. Similarly, at the end of each isometric exercise, do the same in reverse as you disengage from the exercise over a period of between 2 and 3 seconds.

△ Perform the workout on 3 alternate days for your first week of The ISO90™ Course on: Monday / Wednesday / Friday.

△ Take two days of rest over the weekend before starting the workout routine again on the following Monday.

Introductory Optional Cardio

If you wish to perform a basic cardio exercise, then we'd suggest the alternate knee to chest exercise. How many you perform, for how long, and at what pace will all

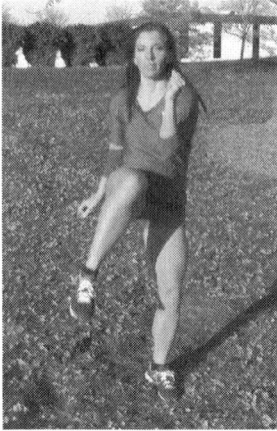

depend upon your basic level of fitness when you start The ISO90™ Course.

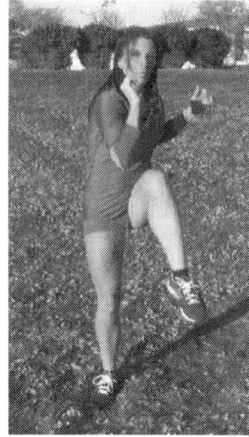

If you're a complete beginner, then it may be that you perform one set of as many as possible in as little as 10 or 20 seconds. However, if you're already fit then you'll be able to perform a great many more, for much longer and at a more intense pace.

Legs - Upper Thighs

Beginner: Iso-Bow® Squat Position Bodyweight Only
Experienced: Iso-Bow® Wall Squat with Resistance

The Squat exercise can be performed in various ways, and to begin with we'll approach it from that of both a basic and intermediary athlete to perform a wall squat.

Stand upright, close to a wall, door, vehicle or any other immovable object to aid with your stability and to help maintain perfect exercise form.

Bend the knees as deeply as comfortably possible

being sure that you only bend your torso at the hips, so that you can keep your back straight and upright at all times.

If you're a complete unfit beginner, then assuming the wall squat position, you may need to place the Iso-Bow® over the top of the thighs, just above the knees.

In this position, instead of providing resistance for the exercise, the Iso-Bow® provides support until your thigh muscles are strong enough to perform the intermediate and advanced exercises later in the course. Once you've assumed the position, then push backwards and upwards using the thigh muscles.

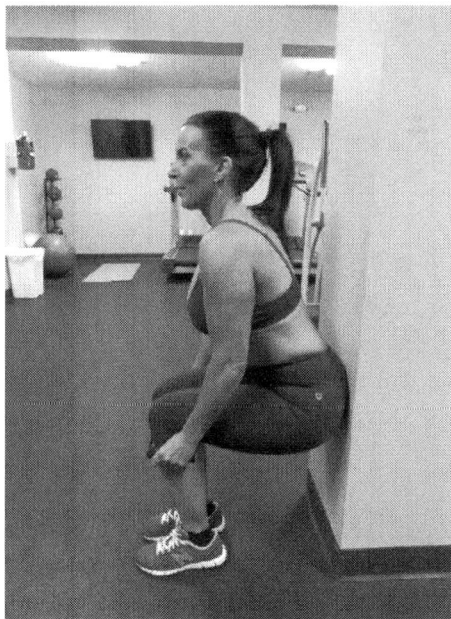

If you're already fit and flexible enough, then perform the more advanced exercise and by placing the Iso-Bow® comfortably around your upper shins just under the knee, so that your shins serve as the resistance anchor point for you to engage the upper thigh muscles during the exercise.

In this wall squat position, grip each Iso-Bow® handle firmly as you attempt to stand up straight by engaging the upper thigh and glute muscles. You'll effectively be pushing back, and up against the wall, in a sort of inverted-upright leg press movement.

Naturally you won't be able to move, but continue to push as intensely as possible while maintaining a perfect mid-squat position at all times during the exercise.

Breathe naturally and deeply in and out for about 10 full breaths, which will take about 1 second per breath. Aim to perform an exercise breathing count of no less than 7 seconds, and for no longer than 10 seconds.

Chest

Iso-Bow® Chest Cross Press Wide

Cross the Iso-Bow® in front of you at chest level,

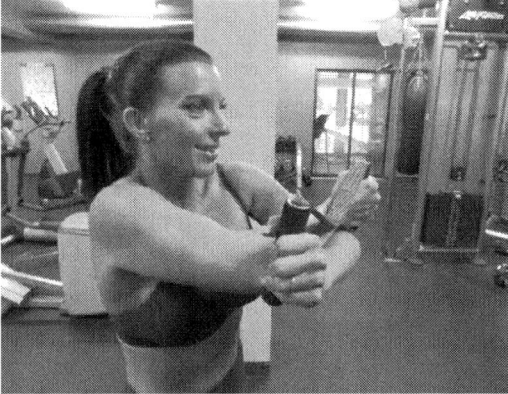

with your arms roughly parallel to the floor, and push in opposing directions sideways to engage your chest muscles.

Breathe naturally and deeply in and out for about 10 full breaths, which will take about 1 second per breath.

Aim to perform an exercise breathing count of no less than 7 seconds, and for no longer than 10 seconds.

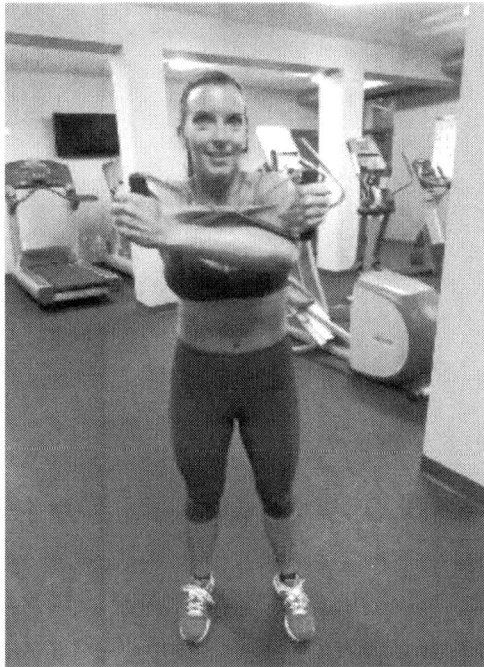

Upper Back

Iso-Bow® Back Power Pull Wide

Hold the Iso-Bow in front of you, with your arms slight bent, and approximately parallel to the floor, and

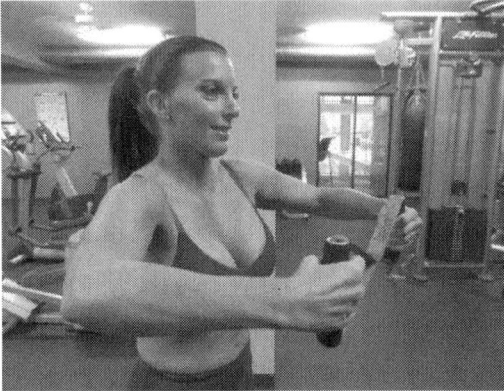

attempt to pull the Iso-Bow apart to engage the upper back muscles.

Breathe naturally and deeply in and out for about 10 full breaths, which will take about 1 second per breath.

Aim to perform an exercise breathing count of no less than 7 seconds, and for no longer than 10 seconds.

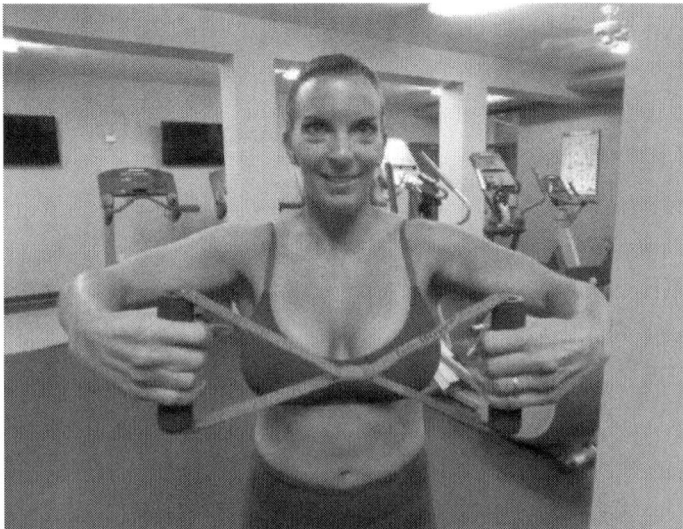

Arms – Biceps and Triceps

Iso-Bow® Biceps and Triceps Cradle Press-Curl (Left Side)

Firstly, you'll exercise the biceps of your right arm, and triceps muscles of your left arm.

Cradle the Iso-Bow with your left hand, gripping the top with your right hand facing up. Grip the cradled side of the Iso-Bow with the left hand facing down.

Keep both elbows close to your body, and with your right arm across the front of you at waist height. In this position, press down with the left hand, and at the same time press up with the right, to engage both the Biceps and Triceps muscles simultaneously.

Breathe naturally and deeply in and out for about 10 full breaths, which will take about 1 second per breath.

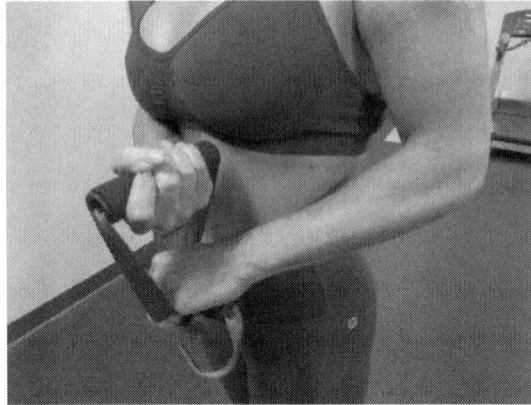

Aim to perform an exercise breathing count of no less than 7 seconds, and for no longer than 10 seconds.

Next, you'll need to perform the same exercise in reverse so that you now engage the biceps of your left arm, and triceps muscles of your right arm.

Iso-Bow® Biceps and Triceps Cradle Press-Curl (Right Side)

Cradle the Iso-Bow® with your right hand, gripping the top with your left hand facing up. Grip the cradled side

of the Iso-Bow with the right hand facing down.

Keep both elbows close to your body, and with your left arm across the front of you at waist height. In this position, press down with the right hand, and at the same time press up with the

left, to engage both the Biceps and Triceps muscles simultaneously.

Breathe naturally and deeply in and out for about 10 full breaths, which will take about 1 second per breath.

Aim to perform an exercise breathing count of no less than 7 seconds, and for no longer than 10 seconds.

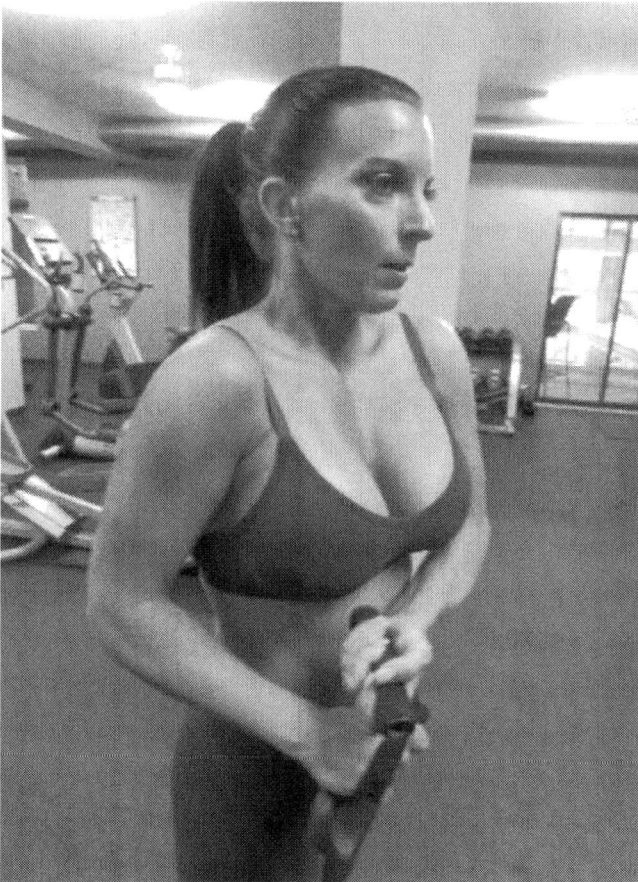

Abdominals

Iso-Bow® Seated Knee Raise and Forward Trunk Curl

Sit on a chair, car seat or bench, place the Iso-Bow® with handles facing downwards, over the top of one knee. Then, curl your body forwards and downwards by contracting the abdominals, and at the same time, raise the knee resisted by the Iso-Bow®.

Perform each exercise for no less than 7 seconds, and for no longer than 10.

Breathe deeply and naturally at all times as you exercise, which will be about 10 full breaths, at a rate of about 1 second per breath. Then repeat the exercise using the other knee.

The ISO90™ Course Week 1 at a Glance

Introductory Optional Cardio

Legs - Upper Thighs

- △ *Beginner: Iso-Bow® Squat Position Bodyweight Only*
- △ *Experienced: Iso-Bow® Wall Squat with Resistance*

Chest

- △ *Iso-Bow® Chest Cross Press Wide*

Upper Back

- △ *Iso-Bow® Back Power Pull Wide*

Arms – Biceps and Triceps

- △ *Iso-Bow® Biceps and Triceps Cradle Press-Curl (Left Side)*
- △ *Iso-Bow® Biceps and Triceps Cradle Press-Curl (Right Side)*

Abdominals

- △ *Iso-Bow® Seated Knee Raise and Forward Trunk Curl*

The ISO90™ Course Week 2

Week 2 Notes

⚠ Slightly increase the intensity used with all exercises, and slightly reduce the amount of rest time between exercises. Apply approximately 60% of your maximum potential intensity to each exercise.

Perform only one 7 second isometric exercise contraction. *(Don't start counting until you've fully applied the desired level of intensity)*

⚠ Before you begin the full isometric contraction part of the exercise, take between 2 and 3 additional seconds to perform Dynamic Flexation™ to help you properly engage the muscles and joints. Similarly, at the end of each isometric exercise, do the same in reverse as you disengage from the exercise over a period of between 2 and 3 seconds.

⚠ Perform the workout on 3 alternate days again for your second week of The ISO90™ Course on: Monday / Wednesday / Friday / and Sunday. However, your next phase for week 3 begins the next day on Sunday, without a weekend of rest.

Introductory Optional Cardio

If you still wish to perform a basic cardio exercise, then we'd suggest the alternate knee to chest exercise. How many you perform, for how long, and at what pace will

66

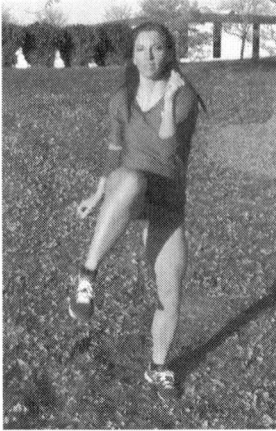

all depend upon your basic level of fitness when you start The ISO90™ Course.

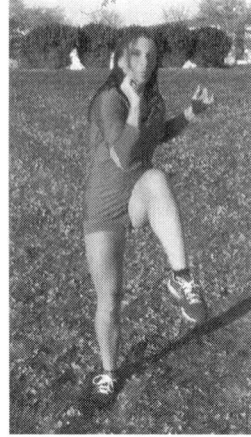

If you're a complete beginner, then it may be that you perform one set of as many as possible in as little as 10 or 20 seconds. However, if you're already fit then you'll be able to perform a great many more, for much longer and at a more intense pace.

Legs – Upper Thighs

Beginner: Iso-Bow® Squat Position Bodyweight Only
Experienced: Iso-Bow® Wall Squat with Resistance

The Squat exercise can be performed in various ways, and to begin with we'll approach it from that of both a basic and intermediary athlete to perform a wall squat.

Stand upright, close to a wall, door, vehicle or any other immovable object to aid with your stability and to help maintain perfect exercise form.

Bend the knees as deeply as comfortably possible being sure that you only bend your torso at the hips, so that you can keep your back straight and upright at all times.

If you're a complete unfit beginner, then assuming the wall squat position, you may need to place the Iso-Bow® over the top of the thighs, just above the knees.

In this position, instead of providing resistance for the exercise, the Iso-Bow® provides support until your thigh muscles are strong enough to perform the intermediate and advanced exercises later in the course. Once you've assumed the position, then push backwards and upwards using the thigh muscles.

If you're already fit and flexible enough, then perform the more advanced exercise and by placing the Iso-Bow® comfortably around your upper shins just under the knee, so that your shins serve as the resistance anchor point for you to engage the upper thigh muscles during the exercise.

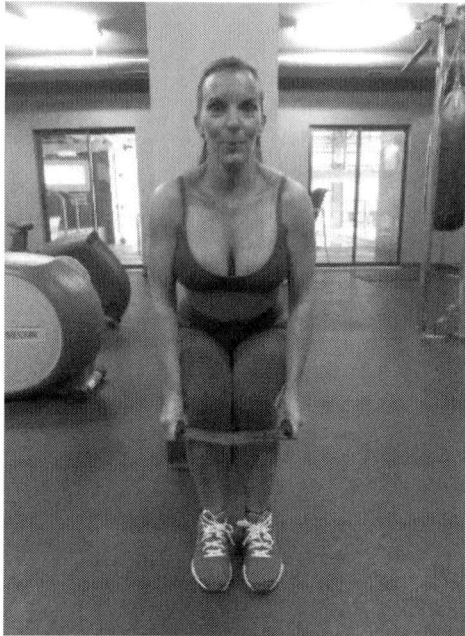

In this wall squat position, grip each Iso-Bow® handle firmly as you attempt to stand up straight by engaging the upper thigh and glute muscles. You'll effectively be pushing back, and up against the wall, in a sort of inverted-upright leg press movement.

Naturally you won't be able to move, but continue to push as intensely as possible while maintaining a perfect mid-squat position at all times during the exercise.

Breathe naturally and deeply in and out for about 10 full breaths, which will take about 1 second per breath. Aim to perform an exercise breathing count of no less than 7 seconds, and for no longer than 10 seconds.

Chest

Iso-Bow® Chest Cross Press Wide

Cross the Iso-Bow® in front of you at chest level, with your arms roughly parallel to the floor, and push in opposing directions sideways to engage your chest muscles.

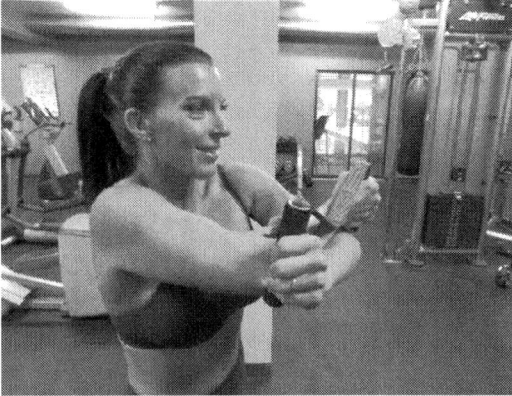

Breathe naturally and deeply in and out for about 10 full breaths, which will take about 1 second per breath.

Aim to perform an exercise breathing count of no less than 7 seconds, and for no longer than 10 seconds.

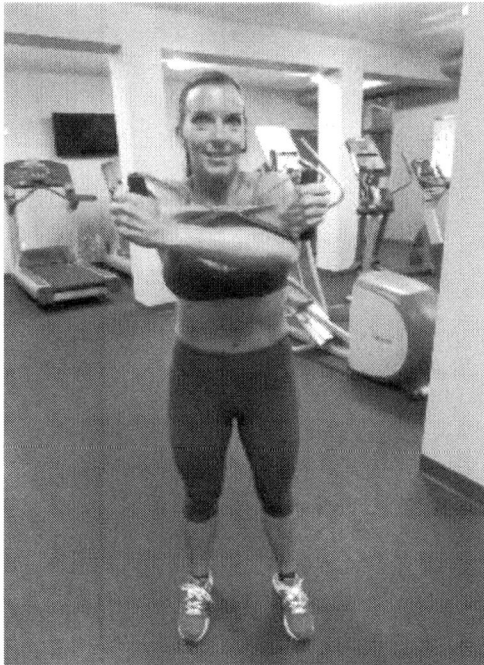

70

Upper Back

Iso-Bow® Seated Knee Row

Sit upright on a solid object such as a chair, car seat or bench, bending forwards only from the hips, and keeping your back straight at all times.

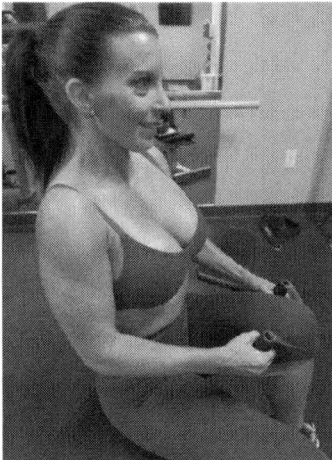

Lift one knee and comfortably wrap the Iso-Bow® around in front of it, pull back with the handles as you engage your upper back muscles, keeping your elbows close to your body as you do so.

Breathe naturally and deeply in and out for about 10 full breaths, which will take about 1 second per breath.

Aim to perform an exercise breathing count of no less than 7 seconds, and for no longer than 10 seconds.

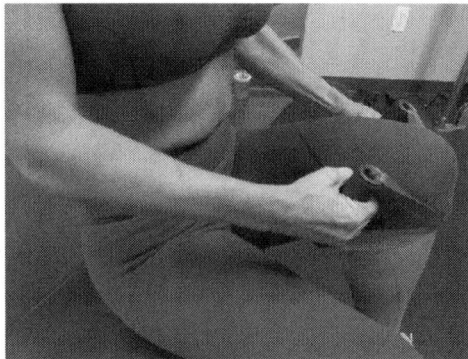

Arms – Biceps and Triceps

Iso-Bow® Biceps and Triceps Cradle Press-Curl (Left Side)

Firstly, you'll exercise the biceps of your right arm, and triceps muscles of your left arm.

Cradle the Iso-Bow with your left hand, gripping the top with your right hand facing up. Grip the cradled side of the Iso-Bow with the left hand facing down.

Keep both elbows close to your body, and with your right arm across the front of you at waist height. In this position, press down with the left hand, and at the same time press up with the right, to engage both the Biceps and Triceps muscles simultaneously.

Breathe
naturally
and deeply
in and out
for about 10
full breaths,
which will
take about 1
second per
breath.

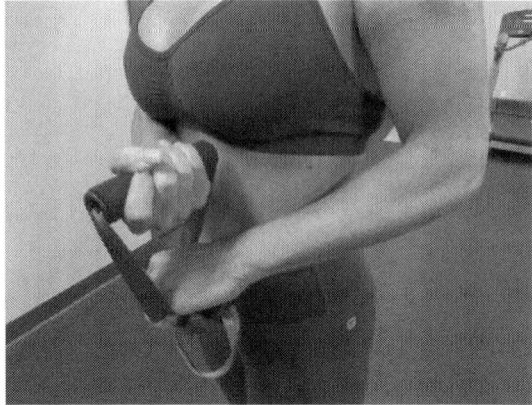

Aim to perform an exercise breathing count of no less than 7 seconds, and for no longer than 10 seconds.

Next, you'll need to perform the same exercise in reverse so that you now engage the biceps of your left arm, and triceps muscles of your right arm.

Iso-Bow® Biceps and Triceps Cradle Press-Curl (Right Side)

Cradle the Iso-Bow® with your right hand, gripping the top with your left hand facing up. Grip the cradled side

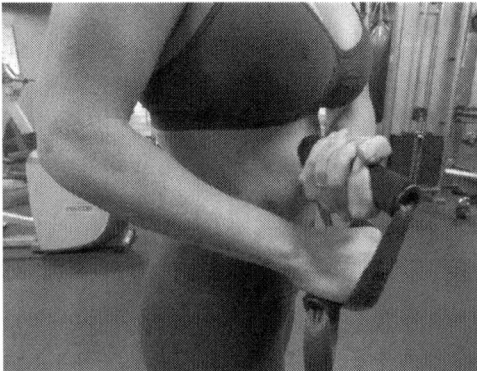

of the Iso-Bow with the right hand facing down.

Keep both elbows close to your body, and with your left arm across the front of you at waist height. In this position, press down with the right hand, and at the same time press up with the

left, to engage both the Biceps and Triceps muscles simultaneously.

Breathe naturally and deeply in and out for about 10 full breaths, which will take about 1 second per breath.

Aim to perform an exercise breathing count of no less than 7 seconds, and for no longer than 10 seconds.

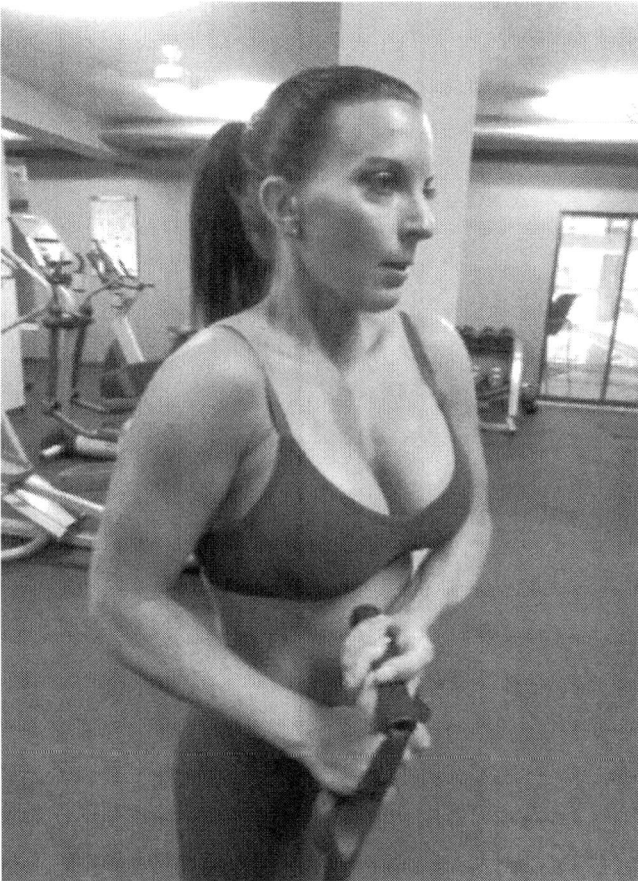

Lower Back

Iso-Bow® Intermediate Back Extension

Stand with your feet shoulder width apart, and with your knees slightly bent. Bend forwards only from the hips as low as you're comfortably able to, hold both handles of an Iso-Bow® downwards towards the floor.

Breathe naturally and deeply in and out for about 10 full breaths, which will take about 1 second per breath. Aim to perform an exercise breathing count of no less than 7 seconds, and for no longer than 10 seconds.

To perform the intermediate exercise, in the same position extend your arms and hold the Iso-Bow® straight

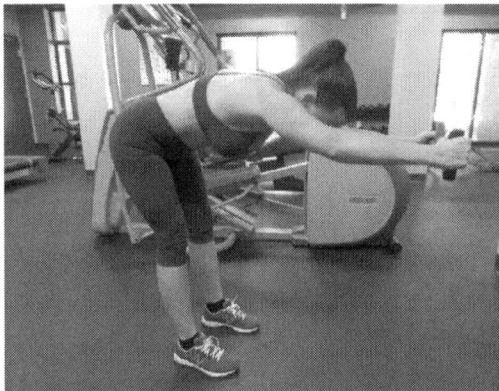

out in front of you as far as you're comfortable to aid both your balance and to increase the resistance on your lower back muscles.

Abdominals

Iso-Bow® Seated Knee Raise and Forward Trunk Curl

Sit on a chair, car seat or bench, place the Iso-Bow® with handles facing downwards, over the top of one knee. Then, curl your body forwards and downwards by contracting the abdominals, and at the same time, raise the knee resisted by the Iso-Bow®.

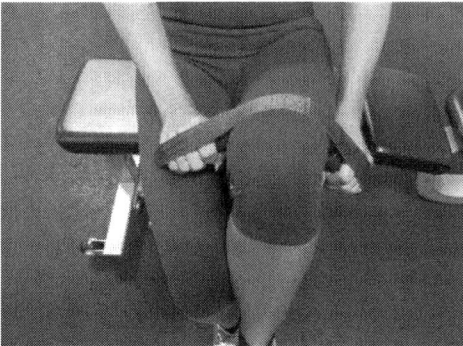

Perform each exercise for no less than 7 seconds, and for no longer than 10.

Breathe deeply and naturally at all times as you exercise, which will be about 10 full breaths, at a rate of about 1 second per breath. Then repeat the exercise using the other knee.

The ISO90™ Course Week 2 at a Glance

Introductory Optional Cardio

Legs – Upper Thighs

- ⚠ *Beginner: Iso-Bow® Squat Position Bodyweight Only*
- ⚠ *Experienced: Iso-Bow® Wall Squat with Resistance*

Chest

- ⚠ *Iso-Bow® Chest Cross Press Wide*

Upper Back

- ⚠ *Iso-Bow® Seated Knee Row*

Arms – Biceps and Triceps

- ⚠ *Iso-Bow® Biceps and Triceps Cradle Press-Curl (Left Side)*
- ⚠ *Iso-Bow® Biceps and Triceps Cradle Press-Curl (Right Side)*

Lower Back

- ⚠ *Iso-Bow® Intermediate Back Extension*

Abdominals

- ⚠ *Iso-Bow® Seated Knee Raise and Forward Trunk Curl*

The ISO90™ Course Week 3

Week 3 Notes

△ Slightly increase the intensity used with all exercises, and slightly reduce the amount of rest time between exercises.

△ Apply a little over approximately 60% of your maximum potential intensity to each exercise.

Perform only one 7 second isometric exercise contraction. *(Don't start counting until you've fully applied the desired level of intensity)*

△ Before you begin the full isometric contraction part of the exercise, take between 2 and 3 additional seconds to perform Dynamic Flexation™ to help you properly engage the muscles and joints. Similarly, at the end of each isometric exercise, do the same in reverse as you disengage from the exercise over a period of between 2 and 3 seconds.

△ Perform the workout on every alternate day: Monday / Wednesday / Friday / Sunday / Tuesday etc.

△ Add 3 new exercises to your routine.

Introductory Optional Cardio

If you wish to perform a basic cardio exercise, then we'd still suggest the alternate knee to chest exercise. How many you perform will depend upon how your overall fitness level is developing.

This will depend upon each individual and range from a burst of one set of 10, up to 4 sets in bursts of 10 intense seconds each.

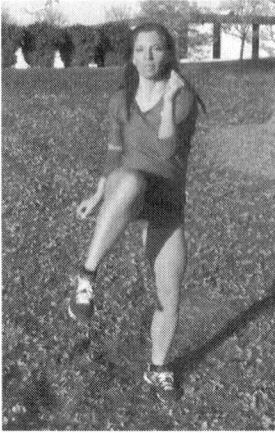

Overall, we'd suggest that you increase the intensity from last week.

Legs – Upper Thighs

Beginner: Iso-Bow® Squat Position Bodyweight Only
Experienced: Iso-Bow® Wall Squat with Resistance

The Squat exercise can be performed in various

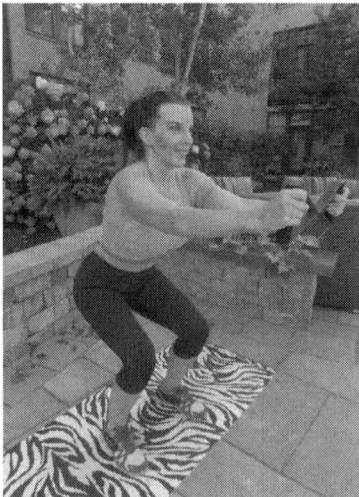

ways, and to begin with we'll approach it from that of both a basic and intermediary athlete to perform a wall squat.

Stand upright, close to a wall, door, vehicle or any other immovable object to aid with your stability and to help maintain perfect exercise form.

Bend the knees as deeply as comfortably possible being sure that you only bend your torso at the hips, so that you can keep your back straight and upright at all times.

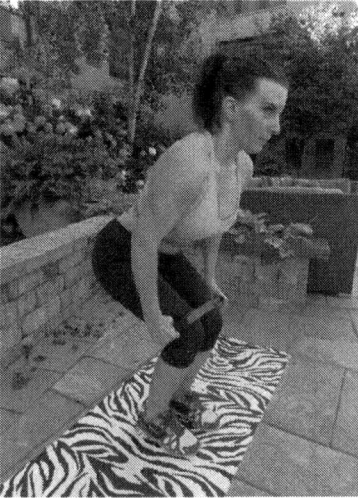

If you're a complete unfit beginner, then assuming the wall squat position, you may need to place the Iso-Bow® over the top of the thighs, just above the knees. In this position, instead of providing resistance for the exercise, the Iso-Bow® provides support until your thigh muscles are strong enough to perform the intermediate and advanced exercises later in the course. Once you've assumed the position, then push backwards and upwards using the thigh muscles.

If you're already fit and flexible enough, then perform the more advanced exercise and by placing the Iso-Bow® comfortably around your upper shins just under the knee, so that your shins serve as the resistance anchor point for you to engage the upper thigh muscles during the exercise.

In this wall squat position, grip each Iso-Bow® handle firmly as you attempt to stand up straight by engaging the upper thigh and glute muscles. You'll effectively be pushing back, and up against the wall, in a sort of inverted-upright leg press movement.

Naturally you won't be able to move, but continue to push as intensely as possible while maintaining a perfect mid-squat position at all times during the exercise.

Breathe naturally and deeply in and out for about 10 full breaths, which will take about 1 second per breath. Aim to perform an exercise breathing count of no less than 7 seconds, and for no longer than 10 seconds.

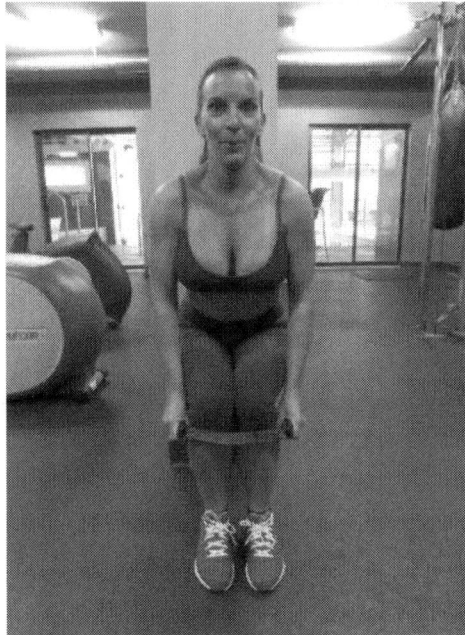

NEW - Calf's

Calf Single Leg Wall Push – Left and Right Leg

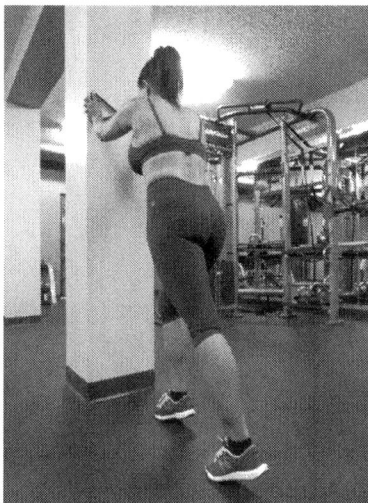

Hold an Iso-Bow® for balance, and place it together with your hands against a wall, a car, a door frame, or any other solid object which is immovable by human muscle power alone.

With one leg behind you in a firm position, and with the ball of your foot on the floor, raise the heel slightly as you engage your calf muscles, pushing against the immovable object.

Breathe naturally and deeply in and out for about 10 full breaths, which will take about 1 second per breath.

Aim to perform an exercise breathing count of no less than 7 seconds, and for no longer than 10 seconds.

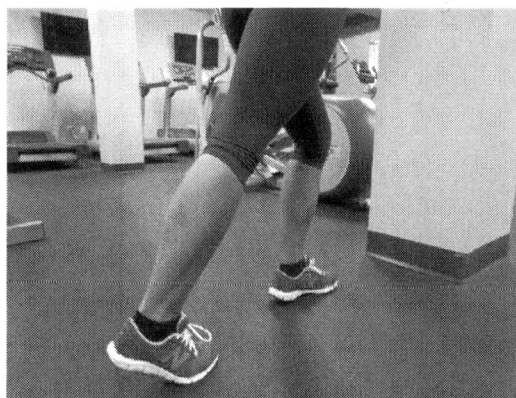

Switch legs and repeat the exercise with the other leg.

Chest

Iso-Bow® Chest Cross Press Wide

Cross the Iso-Bow® in front of you at chest level,

with your arms roughly parallel to the floor, and push in opposing directions sideways to engage your chest muscles.

Breathe naturally and deeply in and out for about 10 full breaths, which will take about 1 second per breath.

Aim to perform an exercise breathing count of no less than 7 seconds, and for no longer than 10 seconds.

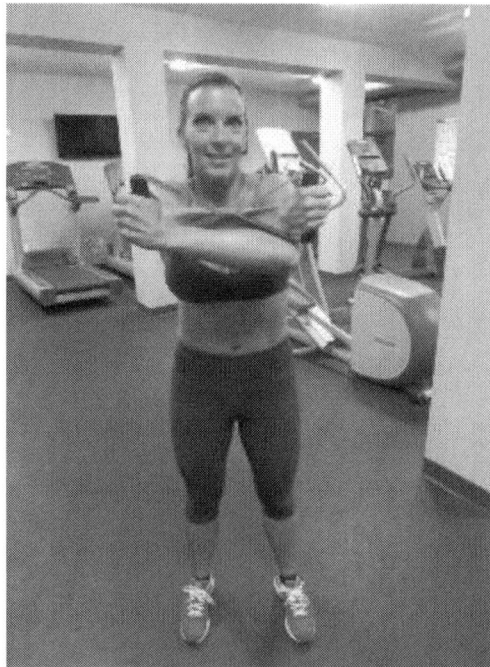

Upper Back

Iso-Bow® Seated Knee Row

Sit upright on a solid object such as a chair, car seat or bench, bending forwards only from the hips, and keeping your back straight at all times.

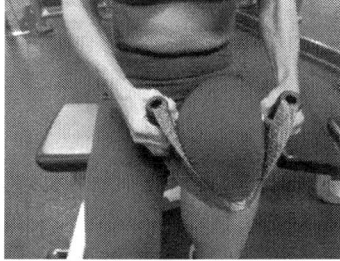

Lift one knee and comfortably wrap the Iso-Bow® around in front of it, pull back with the handles as you engage your upper back muscles, keeping your elbows close to your body as you do so.

Breathe naturally and deeply in and out for about 10 full breaths, which will take about 1 second per breath.

Aim to perform an exercise breathing count of no less than 7 seconds, and for no longer than 10 seconds.

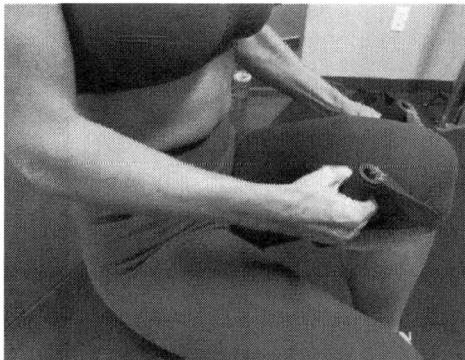

NEW - Shoulders

Iso-Bow® Mid Hold Lateral Pull Apart - AKA Lateral Raise

Hold the Iso-Bow® in both hands, at lap level in front of you, and with your elbows very slightly bent.

In this position, attempt to pull it apart by raising both arms sideways, and engaging the side shoulder muscles as you do so.

Breathe naturally and deeply in and out for about 10 full breaths, which will take about 1 second per breath.

Aim to perform an exercise breathing count of no less than 7 seconds, and for no longer than 10 seconds.

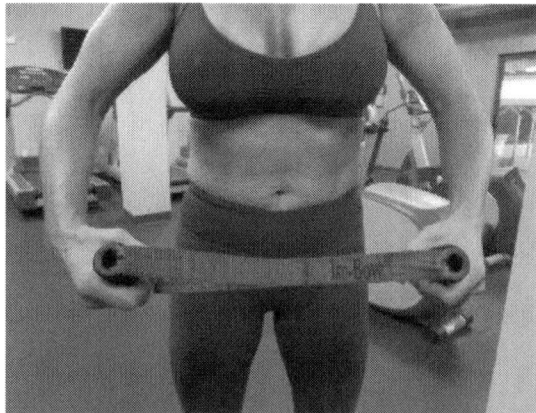

Arms – Biceps and Triceps

Dual Iso-Bow® Foot Loop Biceps Curl

Lean against a solid object, or sit on a chair, car seat or bench, and place the looped ends of two Iso-Bows® around one foot.

Raise that leg slightly until you assume the arm curl position, and then use your leg to provide opposing immovable resistance for your biceps muscles.

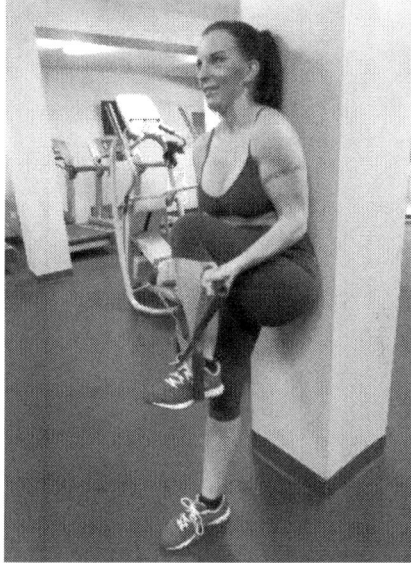

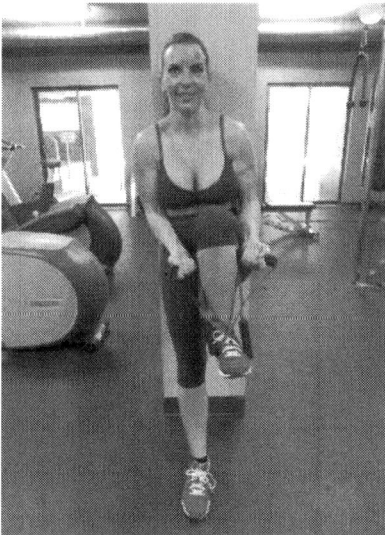

Breathe naturally and deeply in and out for about 10 full breaths, which will take about 1 second per breath.

Aim to perform an exercise breathing count of no less than 7 seconds, and for no longer than 10 seconds.

Iso-Bow® Biceps and Triceps Cradle Press-Curl (Left Side)

Firstly, you'll exercise the biceps of your right arm, and triceps muscles of your left arm.

Cradle the Iso-Bow with your left hand, gripping the top with your right hand facing up. Grip the cradled side of the Iso-Bow with the left hand facing down.

Keep both elbows close to your body, and with your right arm across the front of you at waist height. In this position, press down with the left hand, and at the same time press up with the right, to engage both the Biceps and Triceps muscles simultaneously.

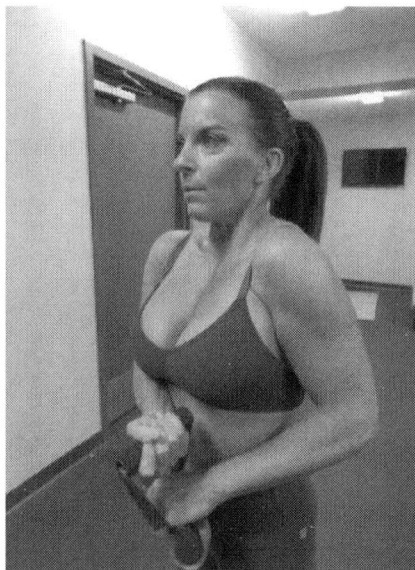

Breathe naturally and deeply in and out for about 10 full breaths, which will take about 1 second per breath.

Aim to perform an exercise breathing count of no less than 7 seconds, and for no longer than 10 seconds.

Next, you'll need to perform the same exercise in reverse so that you now engage the biceps of your left arm, and triceps muscles of your right arm.

Iso-Bow® Biceps and Triceps Cradle Press-Curl (Right Side)

Cradle the Iso-Bow® with your right hand, gripping the top with your left hand facing up. Grip the cradled side of the Iso-Bow with the right hand facing down.

Keep both elbows close to your body, and with your left arm across the front of you at waist height. In this position, press down with the right hand, and at the same time press up with the

left, to engage both the Biceps and Triceps muscles simultaneously.

Breathe naturally and deeply in and out for about 10 full breaths, which will take about 1 second per breath.

Aim to perform an exercise breathing count of no less than 7 seconds, and for no longer than 10 seconds.

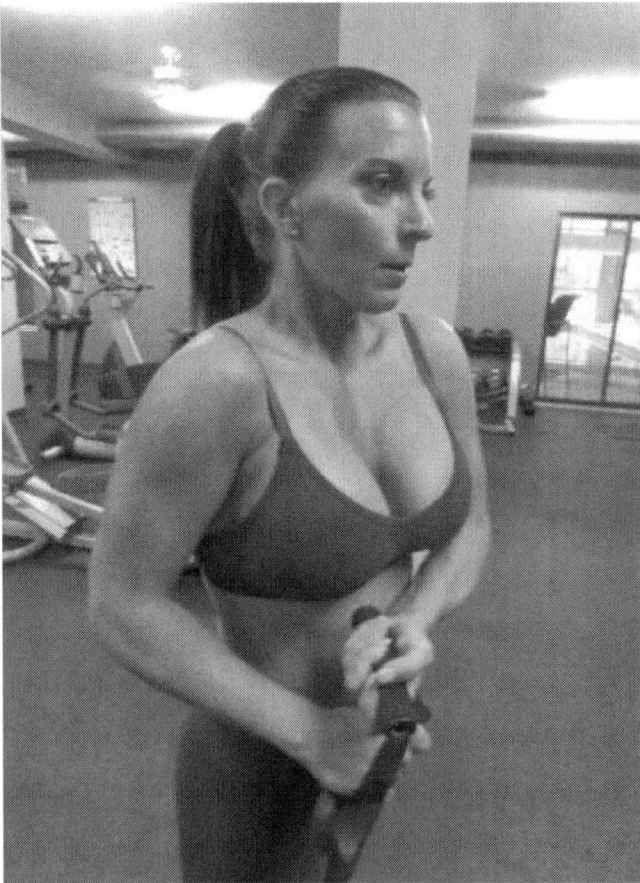

NEW - Lower Back

Dual Iso-Bow® Bent Leg Deadlift

Place the loop handle of both Iso-Bows® around each foot as shown. Hold each handle firmly while maintaining a perfect bent-knee, semi squat position with your back straight at all times, then attempt to slowly stand up straight.

Engage the muscles of the glutes, hamstrings, lower back, thighs, and other core muscles, while the Iso-Bows® secured by your feet prevent any movement from taking place.

Breathe naturally and deeply in and out for about 10 full breaths, which will take about 1 second per breath.

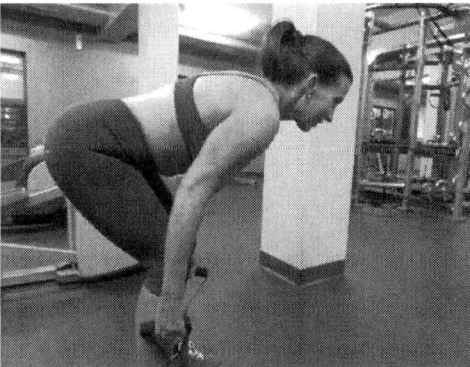

Aim to perform an exercise breathing count of no less than 7 seconds, and for no longer than 10 seconds.

Abdominals

Iso-Bow® Seated Knee Raise and Forward Trunk Curl

Sit on a chair, car seat or bench, place the Iso-Bow® with handles facing downwards, over the top of one knee. Then, curl your body forwards and downwards by contracting the abdominals, and at the same time, raise the knee resisted by the Iso-Bow®.

Perform each exercise for no less than 7 seconds, and for no longer than 10.

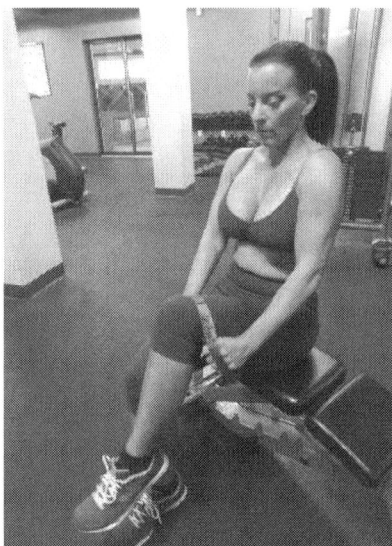

Breathe deeply and naturally at all times as you exercise, which will be about 10 full breaths, at a rate of about 1 second per breath. Then repeat the exercise using the other knee.

The ISO90™ Course Week 3 at a Glance

Introductory Optional Cardio

Legs – Upper Thighs

△ *Beginner: Iso-Bow® Squat Position Bodyweight Only*
△ *Experienced: Iso-Bow® Wall Squat with Resistance*

NEW - Calf's

△ *Calf Single Leg Wall Push – Left and Right Leg*

Chest

△ *Iso-Bow® Chest Cross Press Wide*

Upper Back

△ *Iso-Bow® Seated Knee Row*

NEW - Shoulders

△ *Iso-Bow® Mid Hold Lateral Pull Apart - AKA Lateral Raise*

Arms – Biceps and Triceps

△ *Dual Iso-Bow® Foot Loop Biceps Curl*
△ *Iso-Bow® Biceps and Triceps Cradle Press-Curl (Left Side)*
△ *Iso-Bow® Biceps and Triceps Cradle Press-Curl (Right Side)*

NEW - Lower Back

△ *Dual Iso-Bow® Bent Leg Deadlift*

Abdominals

△ *Iso-Bow® Seated Knee Raise and Forward Trunk Curl*

The ISO90™ Course Week 4

Week 4 Notes

⚠ If possible, slightly increase the intensity used with all exercises, and slightly reduce the amount of rest time between exercises.

⚠ Apply a little over approximately 60% of your maximum potential intensity to each exercise.

Perform only one 7 second isometric exercise contraction. (Don't start counting until you've fully applied the desired level of intensity)

⚠ Before you begin the full isometric contraction part of the exercise, take between 2 and 3 additional seconds to perform Dynamic Flexation™ to help you properly engage the muscles and joints. Similarly, at the end of each isometric exercise, do the same in reverse as you disengage from the exercise over a period of between 2 and 3 seconds.

⚠ Perform the workout EVERY DAY.

⚠ The week starts a completely NEW routine.

Introductory Optional Cardio

If you still wish to perform a basic cardio exercise, then we'd still suggest the alternate knee to chest exercise. How many you perform will depend upon how your overall fitness level is developing as a result of the course.

This will depend upon each Individual and range from a burst of one set of 10, up to 5 sets in bursts of 10 intense seconds each.

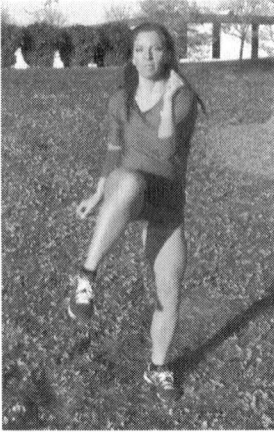

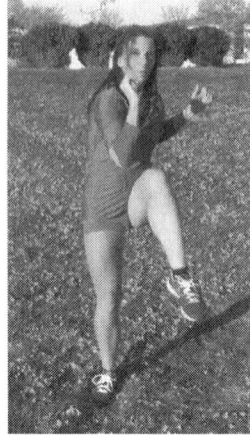

Overall, we'd suggest that you increase the intensity from last week.

Legs – Upper Thighs

Iso-Bow® Forward Lunge - Left and Right Leg

Place the looped ends of two Iso-Bows® around the foot as shown to make a double stirrup. Bend the knee to about 90 degrees, while at the same time move the other leg backwards, with your trailing knee close to the floor, to create a leg-lunge position.

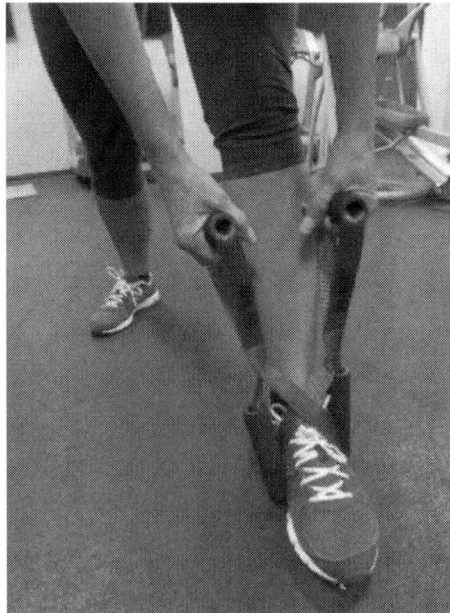

Hold both Iso-Bow® handles firmly, and keeping your body upright and your back straight, use and engage the thigh and glute muscles of your leading leg as you attempt to straighten it and push upwards.

Breathe naturally and deeply in and out for about 10 full breaths, which will take about 1 second per breath.

Aim to perform an exercise breathing count of no less than 7 seconds, and for no longer than 10 seconds. Repeat the exercise with the other leg.

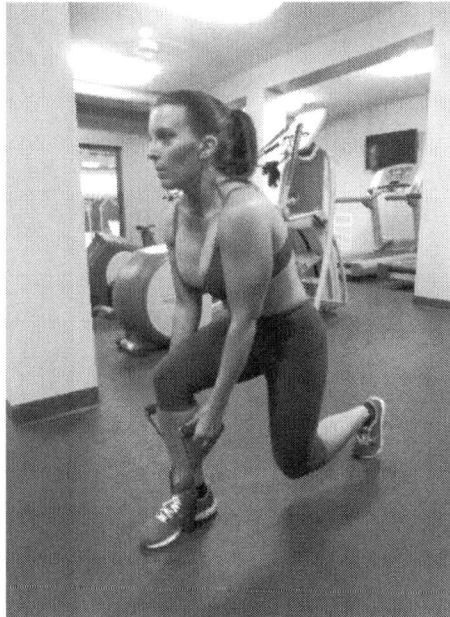

Calf's

Calf Single Leg Wall Push – Left and Right Leg

Hold an Iso-Bow® for balance, and place it together with your hands against a wall, a car, a door frame, or any other solid object which is immovable by human muscle power alone.

With one leg behind you in a firm position, and with the ball of your foot on the floor, raise the heel slightly as you engage your calf muscles, pushing against the immovable object.

Breathe naturally and deeply in and out for about 10 full breaths, which will take about 1 second per breath.

Aim to perform an exercise breathing count of no less than 7 seconds, and for no longer than 10 seconds.

Switch legs and repeat the exercise with the other leg.

Chest

Iso-Bow® Cradle Cross Press

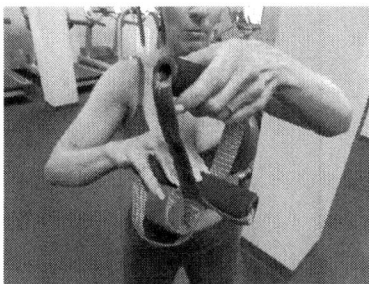

Cradle the Iso-Bow® to make a shorter hand grip, cross it in front of you at chest level, with your arms roughly parallel to the floor, and push in opposing directions sideways to engage your chest muscles.

Breathe naturally and deeply in and out for about 10 full breaths, which will take about 1 second per breath. Aim to perform an exercise breathing count of no less than 7 seconds, and for no longer than 10 seconds.

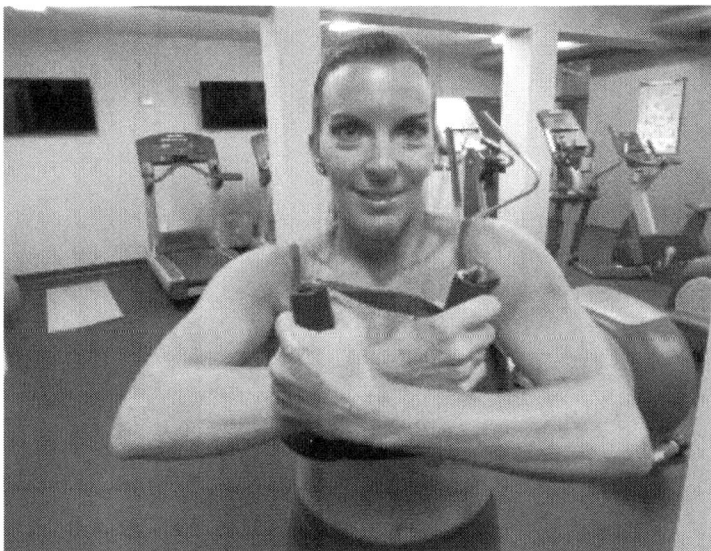

Upper Back

Iso-Bow® Latissimus Overhead Pull Apart

Grip the Iso-Bow® handle, placing the central section comfortably and flat, just above the top of the head. In this position, try to pull your hands apart, engaging the latissimus muscles of the upper back as you do so.

Breathe naturally and deeply in and out for about 10 full breaths, which will take about 1 second per breath. Aim to perform an exercise breathing count of no less than 7 seconds, and for no longer than 10 seconds.

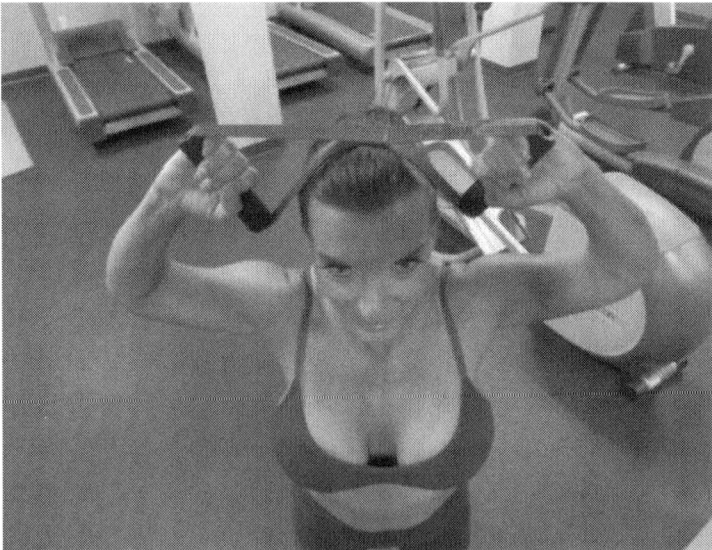

Shoulders

Iso-Bow® Front Raise - Left and Right Arm

Hold each handle of the Iso-Bow® firmly in front of you as shown. Keeping your leading elbow slightly bent, and use the front shoulder muscles to resist the downwards pull of the lower hand and arm.

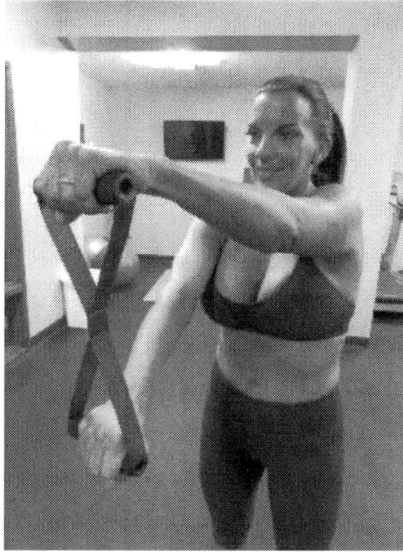

Breathe naturally and deeply in and out for about 10 full breaths, which will take about 1 second per breath.

Aim to perform an exercise breathing count of no less than 7 seconds, and for no longer than 10 seconds.

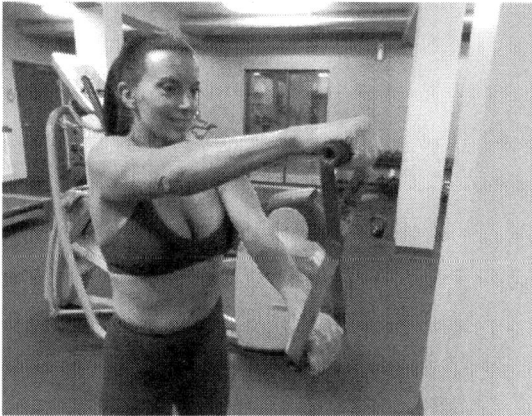

Repeat the exercise on the other side by reversing the hand and arm positions.

Arms - Triceps

Iso-Bow® Triceps Front Press - Left and Right Arm

Hold the Iso-Bow® up to your left shoulder, with your left hand gripping the handle. Hold the other handle

with your right hand facing away from you, keeping your arm at a 90-degree angle.

Engage the triceps muscles of the bent arm, by attempting to push your hand away, against the resistance provided by your left hand, securely holding the Iso-Bow®.

Breathe naturally and deeply in and out for about 10 full breaths, which will take about 1 second per breath.

Aim to perform an exercise breathing count of no less than 7 seconds, and for no longer than 10

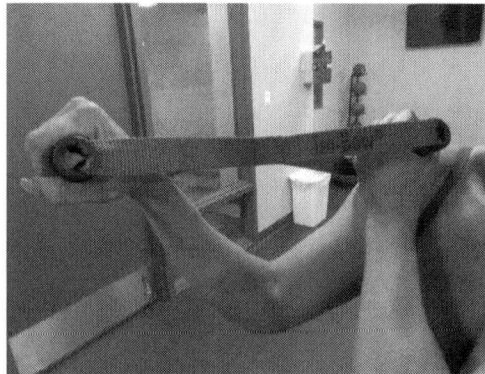

seconds. Repeat on the other side by reversing the action.

Arms - Biceps

Dual Iso-Bow® Foot Loop Biceps Curl

Lean against a solid object, or sit on a chair, car seat or bench, and place the looped ends of two Iso-Bows® around one foot.

Raise that leg slightly until you assume the arm curl position, and then use your leg to provide opposing immovable resistance for your biceps muscles.

Breathe naturally and deeply in and out for about 10 full breaths, which will take about 1 second per breath.

Aim to perform an exercise breathing count of no less than 7 seconds, and for no longer than 10 seconds.

Lower Back

Dual Iso-Bow® Bent Leg Deadlift

Place the loop handle of both Iso-Bows® around each foot as shown. Hold each handle firmly while maintaining a perfect bent-knee, semi squat position with your back straight at all times, then attempt to slowly stand up straight.

Engage the muscles of the glutes, hamstrings, lower back, thighs, and other core muscles, while the Iso-

Bows® secured by your feet prevent any movement from taking place.

Breathe naturally and deeply in and out for about 10 full breaths, which will take about 1 second per breath.

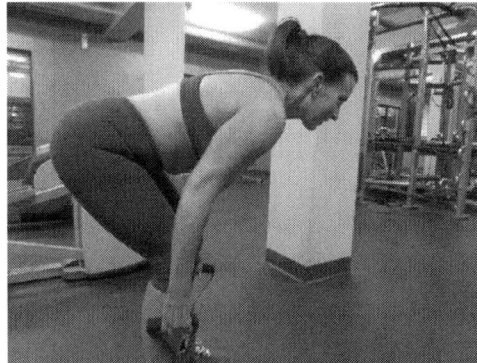

Aim to perform an exercise breathing count of no less than 7 seconds, and for no longer than 10 seconds.

Abdominals

Iso-Bow® Seated Knee Raise and Forward Trunk Curl

Sit on a chair, car seat or bench, place the Iso-Bow®

with handles facing downwards, over the top of one knee. Then, curl your body forwards and downwards by contracting the abdominals, and at the same time, raise the knee resisted by the Iso-Bow®.

Perform each exercise for no less than 7 seconds, and for no longer than 10.

Breathe deeply and naturally at all times as you exercise, which will be about 10 full breaths, at a rate of

about 1 second per breath. Then repeat the exercise using the other knee.

104

The ISO90™ Course Week 4 at a Glance

Introductory Optional Cardio

Legs – Upper Thighs

⚠ *Iso-Bow® Forward Lunge - Left and Right Leg*

Calf's

⚠ *Calf Single Leg Wall Push – Left and Right Leg*

Chest

⚠ *Iso-Bow® Cradle Cross Press*

Upper Back

⚠ *Iso-Bow® Latissimus Overhead Pull Apart*

Shoulders

⚠ *Iso-Bow® Front Raise - Left and Right Arm*

Arms - Triceps

⚠ *Iso-Bow® Triceps Front Press - Left and Right Arm*

Arms - Biceps

⚠ *Dual Iso-Bow® Foot Loop Biceps Curl*

Lower Back

⚠ *Dual Iso-Bow® Bent Leg Deadlift*

Abdominals

⚠ *Iso-Bow® Seated Knee Raise and Forward Trunk Curl*

The ISO90™ Course Week 5

Week 5 Notes

⚠ Increase the intensity used with all exercises, and continue to slightly reduce the amount of rest time between exercises.

⚠ Apply approximately 65% of your maximum potential intensity to each exercise.

Perform only one 7 second isometric exercise contraction. *(Don't start counting until you've fully applied the desired level of intensity)*

⚠ Before you begin the full isometric contraction part of the exercise, take between 2 and 3 additional seconds to perform Dynamic Flexation™ to help you properly engage the muscles and joints. Similarly, at the end of each isometric exercise, do the same in reverse as you disengage from the exercise over a period of between 2 and 3 seconds.

⚠ Perform the workout EVERY DAY, Monday to Friday inclusive, and take Saturday and Sunday as rest days over the weekend.

⚠ Add 1 NEW exercise.

Introductory Optional Cardio

If you still wish to perform a basic cardio exercise, then we'd still suggest the alternate knee to chest exercise. How many you perform will depend upon how your overall fitness level is developing. This will depend upon each individual, and range from a burst of one set of 10, up to 6 sets in bursts of 10 intense seconds each. This week, we'd suggest that you increase the intensity from last week and perform higher intensity bursts of 10 seconds each for 6 sets.

106

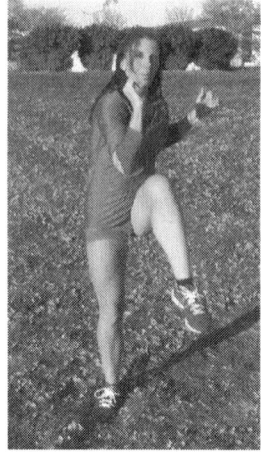

Legs – Upper Thighs

Iso-Bow® Forward Lunge - Left and Right Leg

Place the looped ends of two Iso-Bows® around the foot as shown to make a double stirrup. Bend the knee to about 90 degrees, while at the same time move the other leg backwards, with your trailing knee close to the floor, to create a leg-lunge position.

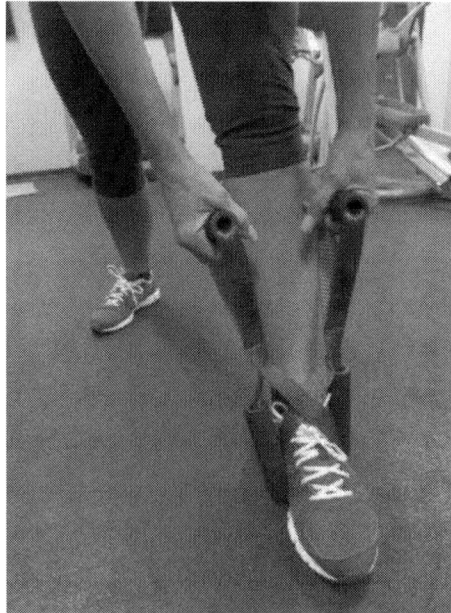

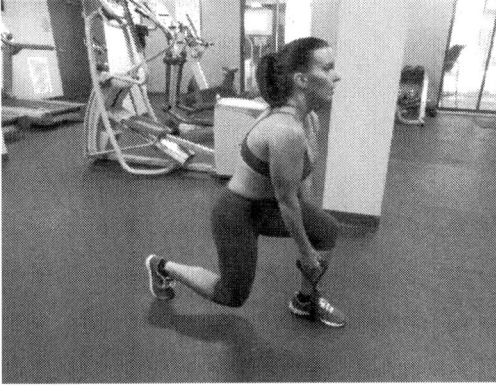

Hold both Iso-Bow® handles firmly, and keeping your body upright and your back straight, use and engage the thigh and glute muscles of your leading leg as you attempt to straighten it and push upwards.

Breathe naturally and deeply in and out for about 10 full breaths, which will take about 1 second per breath.

Aim to perform an exercise breathing count of no less than 7 seconds, and for no longer than 10 seconds. Repeat the exercise with the other leg.

Calf's

Calf Single Leg Wall Push – Left and Right Leg

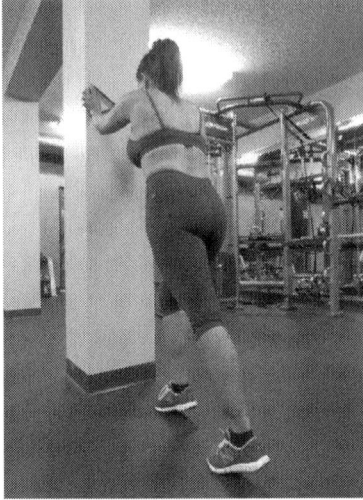

Hold an Iso-Bow® for balance, and place it together with your hands against a wall, a car, a door frame, or any other solid object which is immovable by human muscle power alone.

With one leg behind you in a firm position, and with the ball of your foot on the floor, raise the heel slightly as you engage your calf muscles, pushing against the immovable object.

Breathe naturally and deeply in and out for about 10 full breaths, which will take about 1 second per breath.

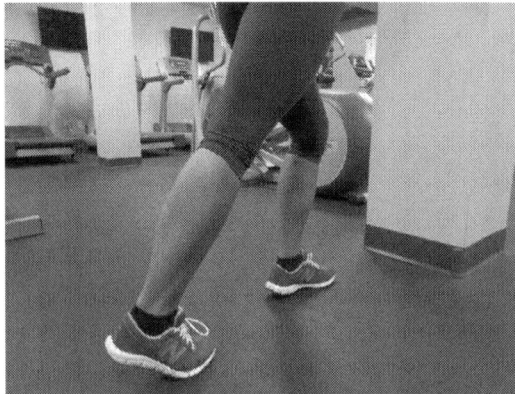

Aim to perform an exercise breathing count of no less than 7 seconds, and for no longer than 10 seconds.

Switch legs and repeat the exercise with the other leg.

Chest

Iso-Bow® Cradle Cross Press

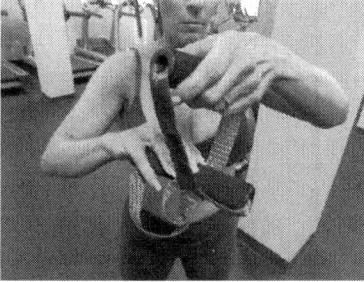

Cradle the Iso-Bow® to make a shorter hand grip, cross it in front of you at chest level, with your arms roughly parallel to the floor, and push in opposing directions sideways to engage your chest muscles.

Breathe naturally and deeply in and out for about 10 full breaths, which will take about 1 second per breath. Aim to perform an exercise breathing count of no less than 7 seconds, and for no longer than 10 seconds.

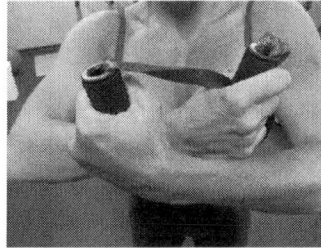

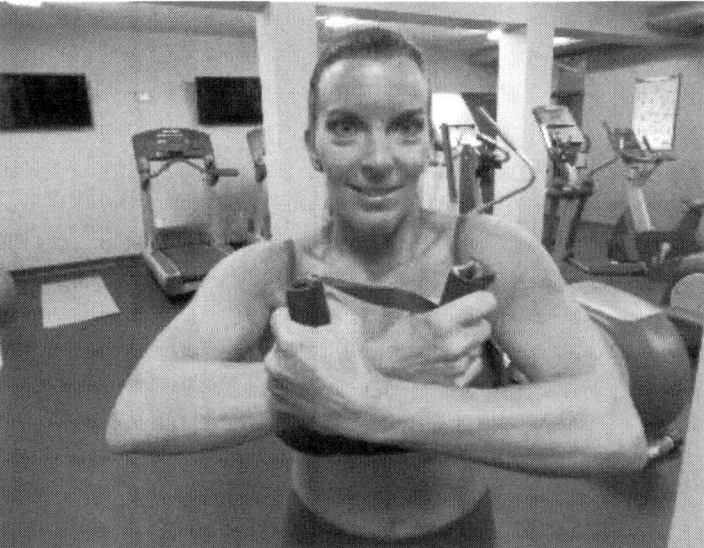

Upper Back

Iso-Bow® Latissimus Overhead Pull Apart

Grip the Iso-Bow® handle, placing the central section comfortably and flat, just above the top of the head. In this position, try to pull your hands apart, engaging the latissimus muscles of the upper back as you do so.

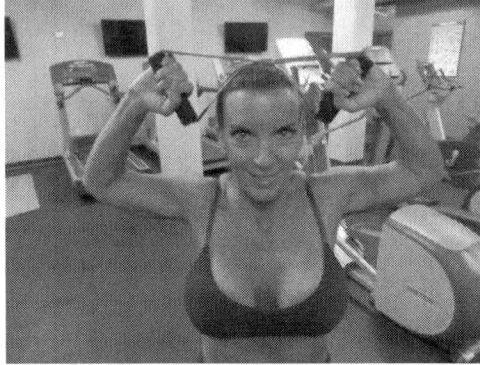

Breathe naturally and deeply in and out for about 10 full breaths, which will take about 1 second per breath. Aim to perform an exercise breathing count of no less than 7 seconds, and for no longer than 10 seconds.

NEW - Iso-Bow® Back Power Pull Wide

Hold the Iso-Bow in front of you, with your arms slight bent, and approximately parallel to the floor, and

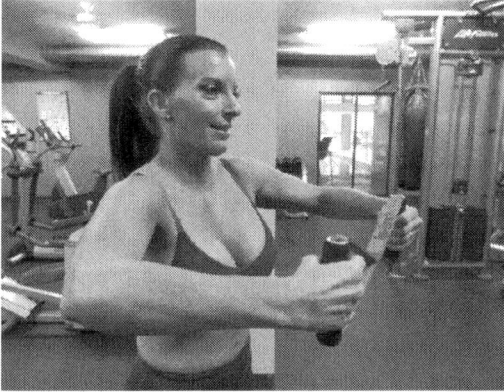

attempt to pull the Iso-Bow apart to engage the upper back muscles.

Breathe naturally and deeply in and out for about 10 full breaths, which will take about 1 second per breath.

Aim to perform an exercise breathing count of no less than 7 seconds, and for no longer than 10 seconds.

Shoulders

Iso-Bow® Front Raise - Left and Right Arm

Hold each handle of the Iso-Bow® firmly in front of you as shown. Keeping your leading elbow slightly bent, and use the front shoulder muscles to resist the downwards pull of the lower hand and arm.

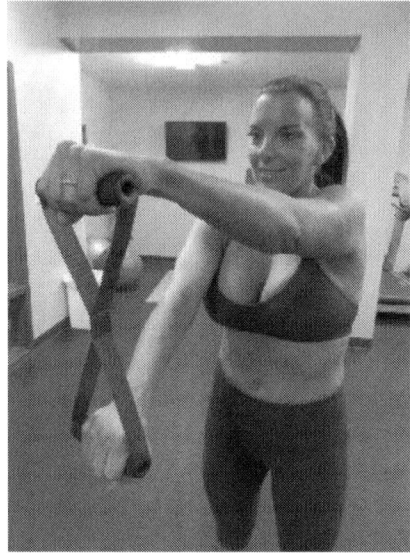

Breathe naturally and deeply in and out for about 10 full breaths, which will take about 1 second per breath.

Aim to perform an exercise breathing count of no less than 7 seconds, and for no longer than 10 seconds.

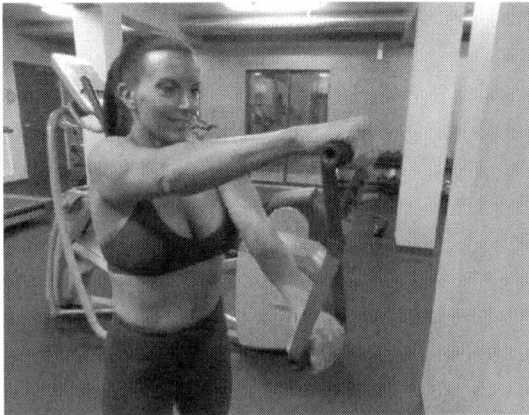

Repeat the exercise on the other side by reversing the hand and arm positions.

Arms - Triceps

Iso-Bow® Triceps Front Press - Left and Right Arm

Hold the Iso-Bow® up to your left shoulder, with your left hand gripping the handle. Hold the other handle

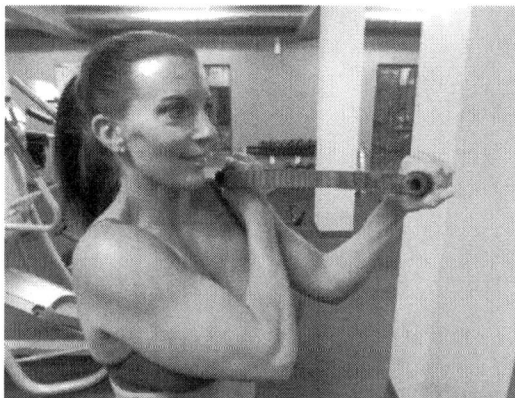

with your right hand facing away from you, keeping your arm at a 90-degree angle.

Engage the triceps muscles of the bent arm, by attempting to push your hand away, against the resistance provided by your left hand, securely holding the Iso-Bow®.

Breathe naturally and deeply in and out for about 10 full breaths, which will take about 1 second per breath.

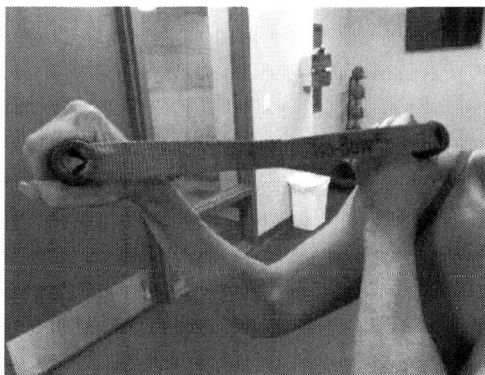

Aim to perform an exercise breathing count of no less than 7 seconds, and for no longer than 10 seconds. Repeat on the other side by reversing the action.

114

Arms - Biceps

Dual Iso-Bow® Foot Loop Biceps Curl

Lean against a solid object, or sit on a chair, car seat or bench, and place the looped ends of two Iso-Bows® around one foot.

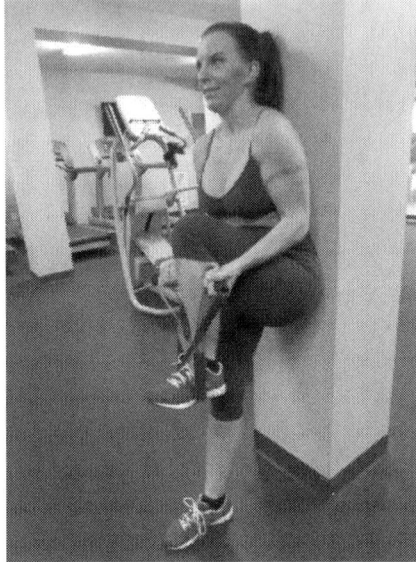

Raise that leg slightly until you assume the arm curl position, and then use your leg to provide opposing immovable resistance for your biceps muscles.

Breathe naturally and deeply in and out for about 10 full breaths, which will take about 1 second per breath.

Aim to perform an exercise breathing count of no less than 7 seconds, and for no longer than 10 seconds.

Lower Back

Dual Iso-Bow® Bent Leg Deadlift

Place the loop handle of both Iso-Bows® around each foot as shown. Hold each handle firmly while maintaining a perfect bent-knee, semi squat position with your back straight at all times, then attempt to slowly stand up straight.

Engage the muscles of the glutes, hamstrings, lower back, thighs, and other core muscles, while the Iso-

Bows® secured by your feet prevent any movement from taking place.

Breathe naturally and deeply in and out for about 10 full breaths, which will take about 1 second per breath.

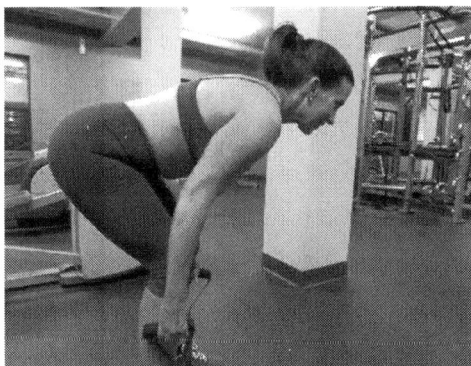

Aim to perform an exercise breathing count of no less than 7 seconds, and for no longer than 10 seconds.

Abdominals

Iso-Bow® Seated Knee Raise and Forward Trunk Curl

Sit on a chair, car seat or bench, place the Iso-Bow® with handles facing downwards, over the top of one knee. Then, curl your body forwards and downwards by contracting the abdominals, and at the same time, raise the knee resisted by the Iso-Bow®.

Perform each exercise for no less than 7 seconds, and for no longer than 10.

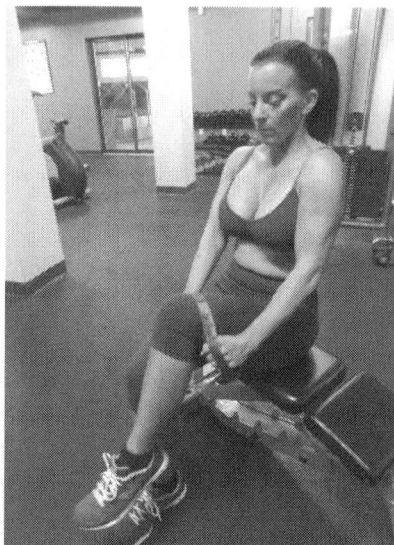

Breathe deeply and naturally at all times as you exercise, which will be about 10 full breaths, at a rate of about 1 second per breath. Then repeat the exercise using the other knee.

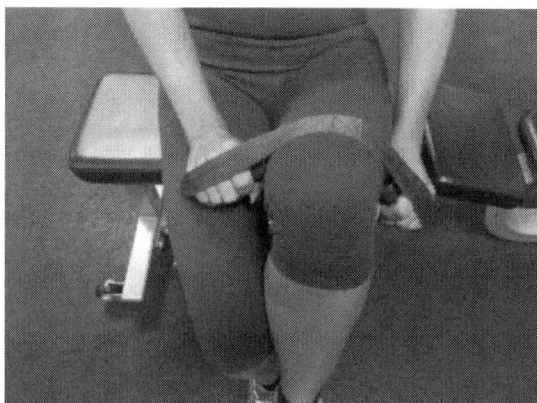

The ISO90™ Course Week 5 at a Glance

Introductory Optional Cardio

Legs – Upper Thighs

⚠ *Iso-Bow® Forward Lunge - Left and Right Leg*

Calf's

⚠ *Calf Single Leg Wall Push – Left and Right Leg*

Chest

⚠ *Iso-Bow® Cradle Cross Press*

Upper Back

⚠ *Iso-Bow® Latissimus Overhead Pull Apart*

⚠ *NEW - Iso-Bow® Back Power Pull Wide*

Shoulders

⚠ *Iso-Bow® Front Raise - Left and Right Arm*

Arms - Triceps

⚠ *Iso-Bow® Triceps Front Press - Left and Right Arm*

Arms - Biceps

⚠ *Dual Iso-Bow® Foot Loop Biceps Curl*

Lower Back

⚠ *Dual Iso-Bow® Bent Leg Deadlift*

Abdominals

⚠ *Iso-Bow® Seated Knee Raise and Forward Trunk Curl*

The ISO90™ Course Week 6

Week 6 Notes

⚠ Continue to try and slightly increase the intensity used with all exercises, while slightly reducing the amount of rest time between exercises.

⚠ Apply approximately 65% of your maximum potential intensity to each exercise.

Perform only one 7 second isometric exercise contraction. *(Don't start counting until you've fully applied the desired level of intensity)*

⚠ Before you begin the full isometric contraction part of the exercise, take between 2 and 3 additional seconds to perform Dynamic Flexation™ to help you properly engage the muscles and joints. Similarly, at the end of each isometric exercise, do the same in reverse as you disengage from the exercise over a period of between 2 and 3 seconds.

⚠ Perform the workout EVERY DAY, Monday to Friday inclusive, and take Saturday and Sunday as rest days over the weekend.

⚠ Add 1 NEW exercise.

Introductory Optional Cardio

If still you wish to perform a basic cardio exercise, then we'd still suggest the alternate knee to chest exercise. How many you perform will depend upon how your overall fitness level is developing. This will depend upon each individual and range from a burst of one set of 10, up to 6 sets in bursts of 10 intense seconds each. This week, we'd suggest that you increase the intensity from last week and perform higher intensity bursts of 10 seconds each for 6 sets.

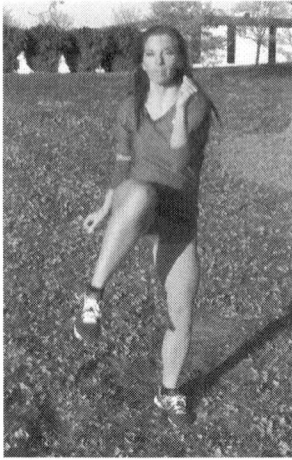

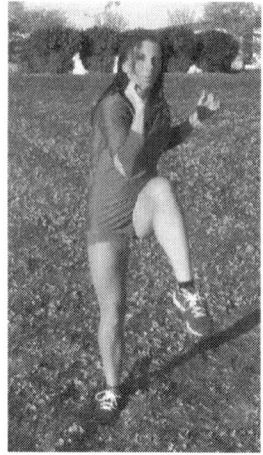

Legs – Upper Thighs

Iso-Bow® Forward Lunge - Left and Right Leg

Place the looped ends of two Iso-Bows® around the foot as shown to make a double stirrup. Bend the knee to about 90 degrees, while at the same time move the other leg backwards, with your trailing knee close to the floor, to create a leg-lunge position.

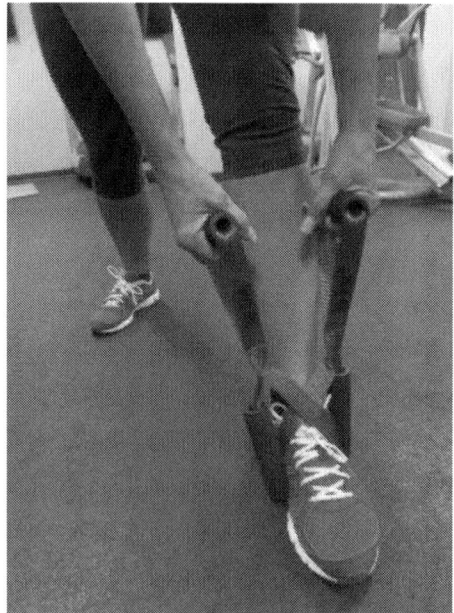

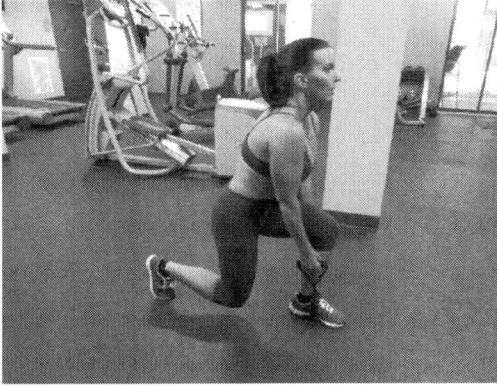

Hold both Iso-Bow® handles firmly, and keeping your body upright and your back straight, use and engage the thigh and glute muscles of your leading leg as you attempt to straighten it and push upwards.

Breathe naturally and deeply in and out for about 10 full breaths, which will take about 1 second per breath.

Aim to perform an exercise breathing count of no less than 7 seconds, and for no longer than 10 seconds. Repeat the exercise with the other leg.

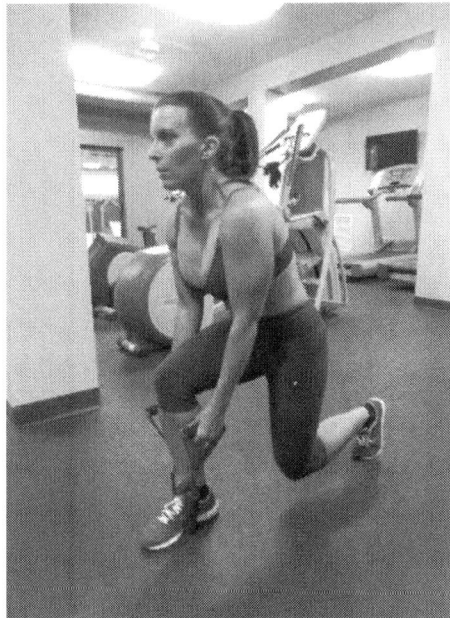

Calf's

Calf Single Leg Wall Push – Left and Right Leg

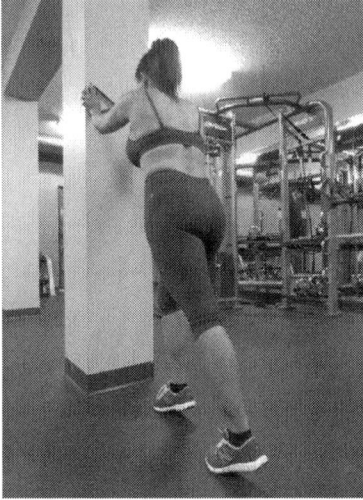

Hold an Iso-Bow® for balance, and place it together with your hands against a wall, a car, a door frame, or any other solid object which is immovable by human muscle power alone.

With one leg behind you in a firm position, and with the ball of your foot on the floor, raise the heel slightly as you engage your calf muscles, pushing against the immovable object.

Breathe naturally and deeply in and out for about 10 full breaths, which will take about 1 second per breath.

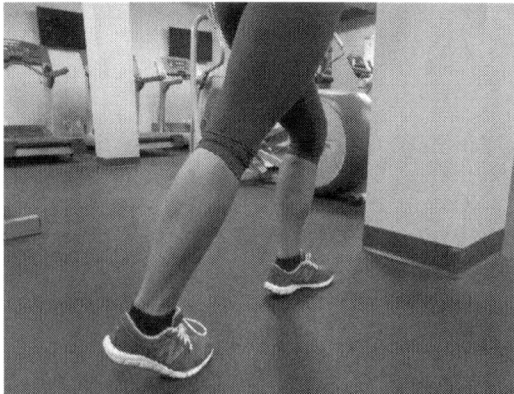

Aim to perform an exercise breathing count of no less than 7 seconds, and for no longer than 10 seconds.

Switch legs and repeat the exercise with the other leg.

Chest

Iso-Bow® Cradle Cross Press

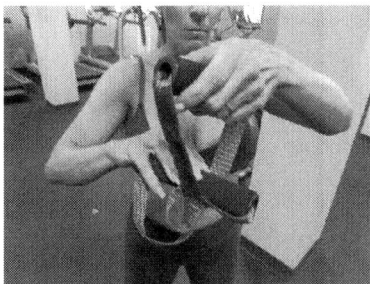

Cradle the Iso-Bow® to make a shorter hand grip, cross it in front of you at chest level, with your arms roughly parallel to the floor, and push in opposing directions sideways to engage your chest muscles.

Breathe naturally and deeply in and out for about 10 full breaths, which will take about 1 second per breath. Aim to perform an exercise breathing count of no less than

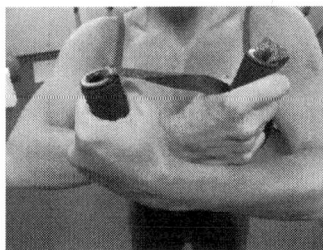

7 seconds, and for no longer than 10 seconds.

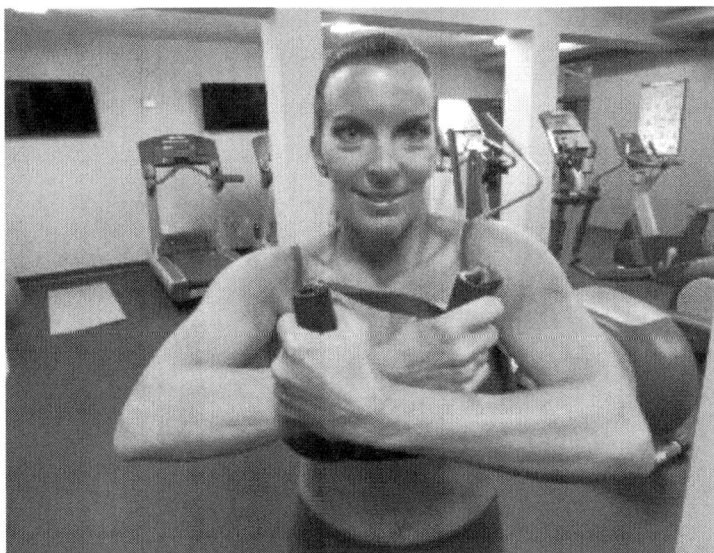

Upper Back

Iso-Bow® Latissimus Overhead Pull Apart

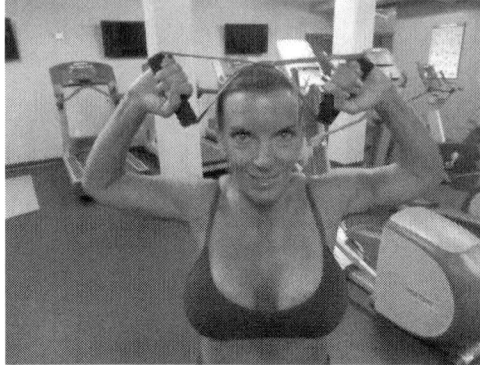

Grip the Iso-Bow® handle, placing the central section comfortably and flat, just above the top of the head. In this position, try to pull your hands apart, engaging the latissimus muscles of the upper back as you do so.

Breathe naturally and deeply in and out for about 10 full breaths, which will take about 1 second per breath. Aim to perform an exercise breathing count of no less than 7 seconds, and for no longer than 10 seconds.

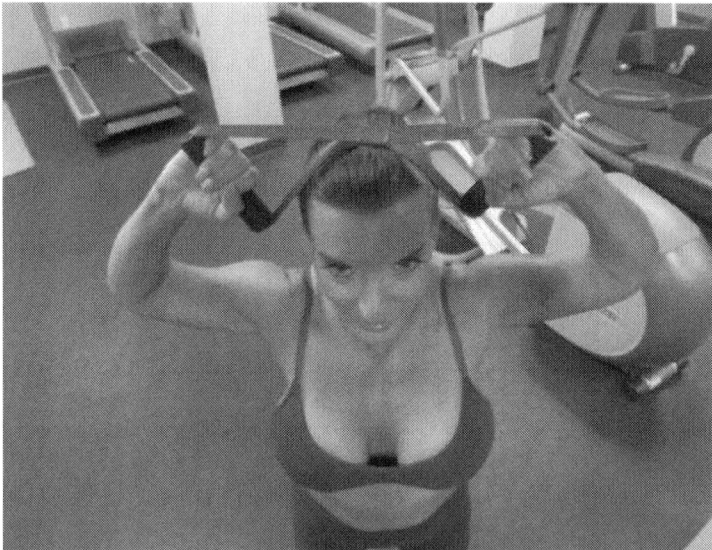

Iso-Bow® Back Power Pull Wide

Hold the Iso-Bow in front of you, with your arms slight bent, and approximately parallel to the floor, and attempt to pull the Iso-Bow apart to engage the upper back muscles.

Breathe naturally and deeply in and out for about 10 full breaths, which will take about 1 second per breath.

Aim to perform an exercise breathing count of no less than 7 seconds, and for no longer than 10 seconds.

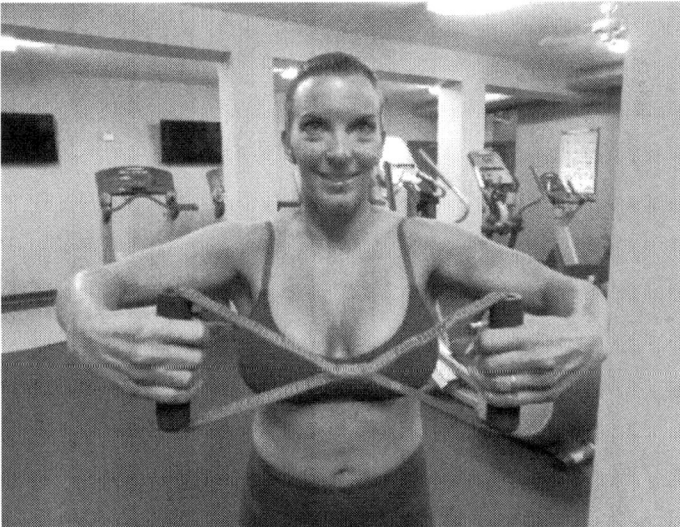

Shoulders

Iso-Bow® Front Raise - Left and Right Arm

Hold each handle of the Iso-Bow® firmly in front of you as shown. Keeping your leading elbow slightly bent, and use the front shoulder muscles to resist the downwards pull of the lower hand and arm.

Breathe naturally and deeply in and out for about 10 full breaths, which will take about 1 second per breath.

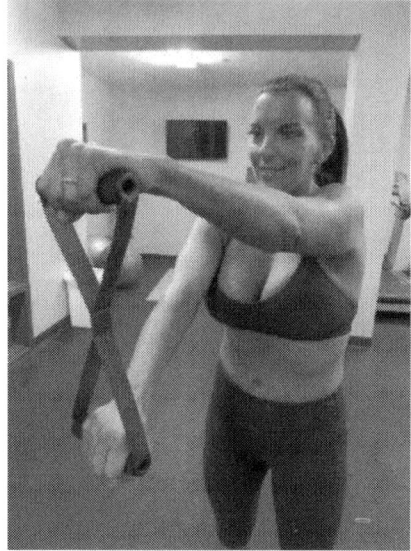

Aim to perform an exercise breathing count of no less than 7 seconds, and for no longer than 10 seconds.

Repeat the exercise on the other side by reversing the hand and arm positions.

Arms - Triceps

Iso-Bow® Triceps Front Press - Left and Right Arm

Hold the Iso-Bow® up to your left shoulder, with your left hand gripping the handle. Hold the other handle

with your right hand facing away from you, keeping your arm at a 90-degree angle.

Engage the triceps muscles of the bent arm, by attempting to push your hand away, against the resistance provided by your left hand, securely holding the Iso-Bow®.

Breathe naturally and deeply in and out for about 10 full breaths, which will take about 1 second per breath.

Aim to perform an exercise breathing count of no less than 7 seconds, and for no longer than 10 seconds. Repeat on the other side by reversing the action.

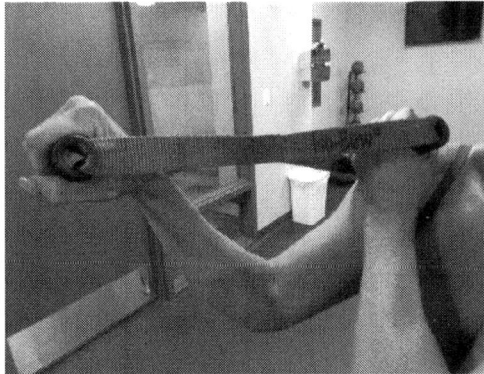

Arms - Biceps

Dual Iso-Bow® Foot Loop Biceps Curl

Lean against a solid object, or sit on a chair, car seat or bench, and place the looped ends of two Iso-Bows® around one foot.

Raise that leg slightly until you assume the arm curl position, and then use your leg to provide opposing immovable resistance for your biceps muscles.

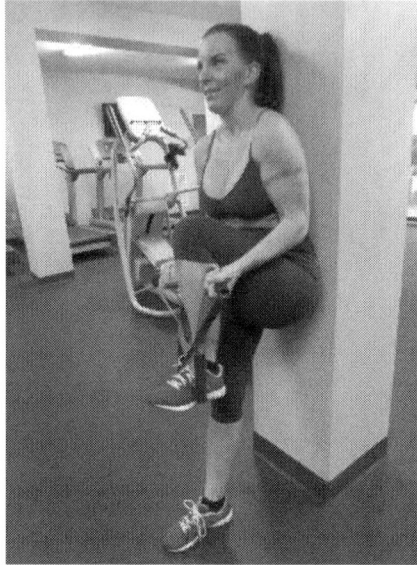

Breathe naturally and deeply in and out for about 10 full breaths, which will take about 1 second per breath.

Aim to perform an exercise breathing count of no less than 7 seconds, and for no longer than 10 seconds.

Lower Back

Dual Iso-Bow® Bent Leg Deadlift

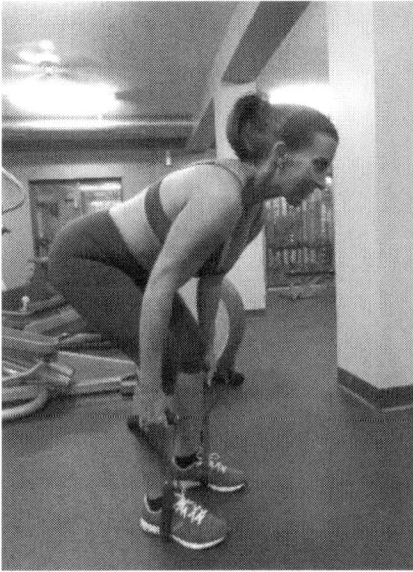

Place the loop handle of both Iso-Bows® around each foot as shown. Hold each handle firmly while maintaining a perfect bent-knee, semi squat position with your back straight at all times, then attempt to slowly stand up straight.

Engage the muscles of the glutes, hamstrings, lower back, thighs, and other core muscles,

while the Iso-Bows® secured by your feet prevent any movement from taking place.

Breathe naturally and deeply in and out for about 10 full breaths, which will take about 1 second per breath.

Aim to perform an exercise breathing count of no less than 7 seconds, and for no longer than 10 seconds.

Abdominals

Iso-Bow® Seated Knee Raise and Forward Trunk Curl

Sit on a chair, car seat or bench, place the Iso-Bow® with handles facing downwards, over the top of one knee. Then, curl your body forwards and downwards by contracting the abdominals, and at the same time, raise the knee resisted by the Iso-Bow®.

Perform each exercise for no less than 7 seconds, and for no longer than 10.

Breathe deeply and naturally at all times as you exercise, which will be about 10 full breaths, at a rate of about 1 second per breath. Then repeat the exercise using the other knee.

131

NEW - Iso-Bow® Kneeling Side Bend
(Iso-Bow® Loop Secured Under Each Knee)

Kneel on the floor with your legs about shoulder width apart, and place the open loop of an Iso-Bow® comfortably under each knee so that the handle will be secured by your kneeling leg.

Keeping your hips upright and in the neutral position, bend sideways until you can hold one Iso-Bow® handle. In that position, use your abdominal oblique muscles of your opposite side to attempt to pull you in an upright direction, naturally you won't be able to move as you apply resistance.

Repeat the exercise on the other side and be sure to never hold both Iso-Bow® handles at the same time.

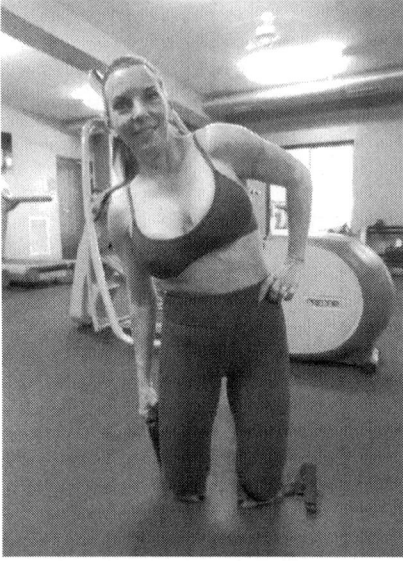

Breathe naturally and deeply in and out for about 10 full breaths, which will take about 1 second per breath. Aim to perform an exercise breathing count of no less than 7 seconds, and for no longer than 10 seconds.

The ISO90™ Course Week 6 at a Glance

Introductory Optional Cardio

Legs – Upper Thighs

⚠ *Iso-Bow® Forward Lunge - Left and Right Leg*

Calf's

⚠ *Calf Single Leg Wall Push – Left and Right Leg*

Chest

⚠ *Iso-Bow® Cradle Cross Press*

Upper Back

⚠ *Iso-Bow® Latissimus Overhead Pull Apart*
⚠ *Iso-Bow® Back Power Pull Wide*

Shoulders

⚠ *Iso-Bow® Front Raise - Left and Right Arm*

Arms - Triceps

⚠ *Iso-Bow® Triceps Front Press - Left and Right Arm*

Arms - Biceps

⚠ *Dual Iso-Bow® Foot Loop Biceps Curl*

Lower Back

⚠ *Dual Iso-Bow® Bent Leg Deadlift*

Abdominals

⚠ *Iso-Bow® Seated Knee Raise and Forward Trunk Curl*
⚠ *NEW - Iso-Bow® Kneeling Side Bend (Iso-Bow® Loop Secured Under Each Knee)*

The ISO90™ Course Week 7

Week 7 Notes

⚠ Increase the intensity used with all exercises, and continue to try to reduce the amount of rest time between exercises.

⚠ Apply approximately 75% of your maximum potential intensity to each exercise.

Perform only one 7 second isometric exercise contraction. *(Don't start counting until you've fully applied the desired level of intensity)*

⚠ Before you begin the full isometric contraction part of the exercise, take between 2 and 3 additional seconds to perform Dynamic Flexation™ to help you properly engage the muscles and joints. Similarly, at the end of each isometric exercise, do the same in reverse as you disengage from the exercise over a period of between 2 and 3 seconds.

⚠ Perform the workout EVERY DAY, Monday to Friday inclusive, and take Saturday and Sunday as rest days over the weekend.

⚠ NEW Technique – Supersets.

Legs – Quadriceps and Hamstring Superset

Iso-Bow® Leg Extension – Single Leg - Left and Right Leg

Sit on a chair, car seat or bench, raise one knee and place the Iso-Bow® comfortably around the lower part of your leg, close to your foot.

Hold the handles firmly, keep your back straight, bending only from the hips, and lean back slightly as you try to raise your leg and push it forwards, keeping your toes upwards at all times.

Breathe naturally and deeply in and out for about 10 full breaths, which will take about 1 second per breath.

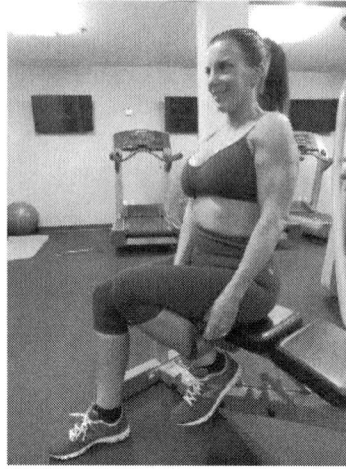

Aim to perform an exercise breathing count of no less than 7 seconds, and for no longer than 10 seconds. Switch legs and repeat the exercise with the other leg.

Iso-Bow® Hamstring Seated Curl – Left and Right Leg

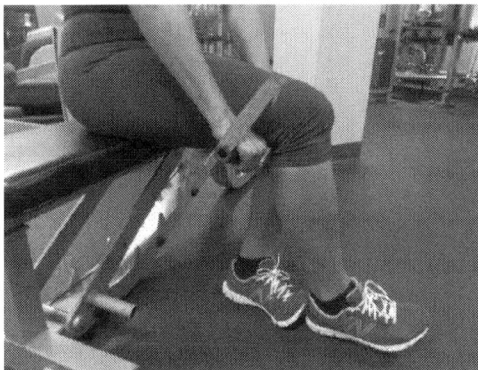

Sit on a chair, car seat or bench, and push the Iso-Bow® comfortably down over one leg to help prevent it from raising up during the exercise.

Place one foot directly in front of the other, so the heel of the leading foot is touching the toes of your rear foot, and turn up the toes to create a firmer connection.

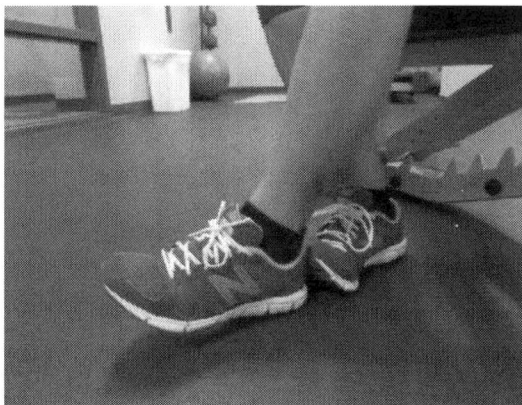

Try to draw back the leading foot by engaging the hamstring muscles of the rear upper thigh.

Breathe naturally and deeply in and out for about 10 full breaths, which will take about 1 second per breath.

Aim to perform an exercise breathing count of no less than 7 seconds, and for no longer than 10 seconds. Repeat the exercise for the other leg, by swapping the leg and foot positions.

Calf's

Calf Single Leg Wall Push – Left and Right Leg

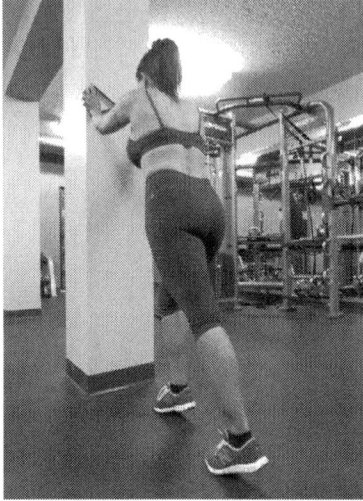

Hold an Iso-Bow® for balance, and place it together with your hands against a wall, a car, a door frame, or any other solid object which is immovable by human muscle power alone.

With one leg behind you in a firm position, and with the ball of your foot on the floor, raise the heel slightly as you engage your calf muscles, pushing against the immovable object.

Breathe naturally and deeply in and out for about 10 full breaths, which will take about 1 second per breath.

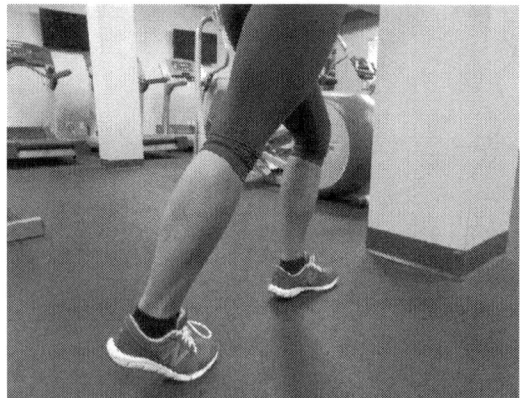

Aim to perform an exercise breathing count of no less than 7 seconds, and for no longer than 10 seconds.

Switch legs and repeat the exercise with the other leg.

Upper Back and Chest Superset

Iso-Bow® Upper Back Seated Knee Brace Row

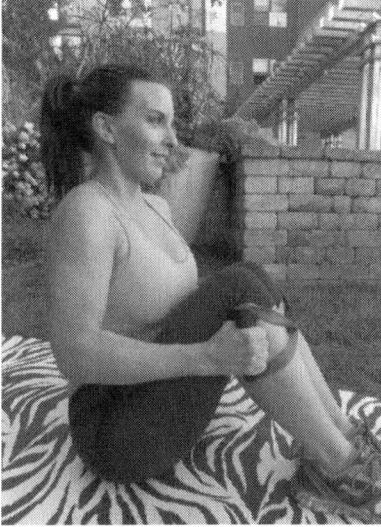

Sit upright on the floor with your feet under a secure object that won't tip over, bending forwards only from the hips, and keeping your back straight at all times.

Wrap the Iso-Bow® comfortably around both knees, and pull back with each handle to engage your upper back muscles, keeping your elbows close to your body as you do so.

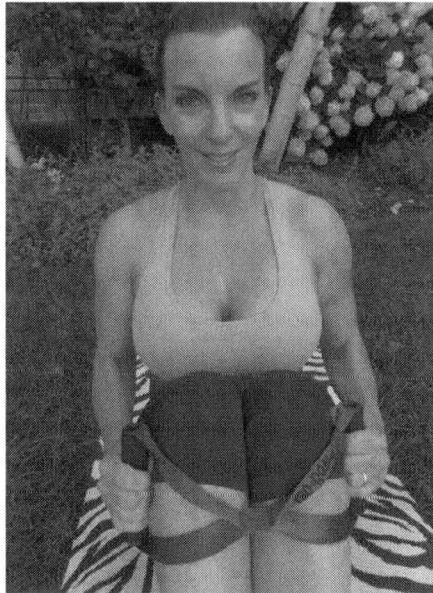

Breathe naturally and deeply in and out for about 10 full breaths, which will take about 1 second per breath.

Aim to perform an exercise breathing count of no less than 7 seconds, and for no longer than 10 seconds.

Iso-Bow® Chest Press and Upper Back Row - Left and Right

With one arm in front of you roughly parallel to the floor, push one end of the Iso-Bow® forwards, and at the same time pull the other handle backwards, keep the elbows of both arms slightly bent at all times.

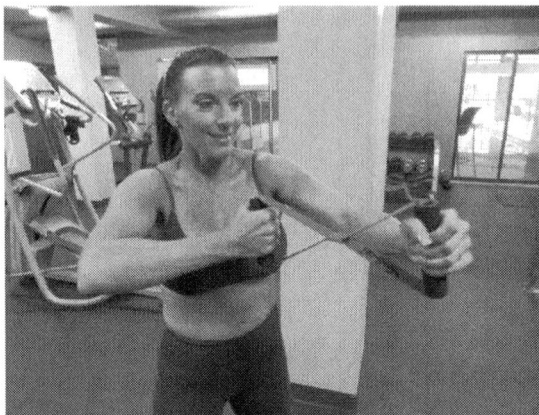

Breathe naturally and deeply in and out for about 10 full breaths, which will take about 1 second per breath.

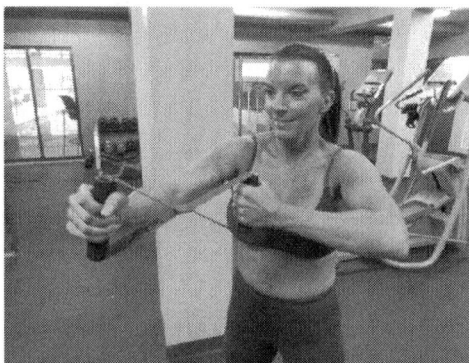

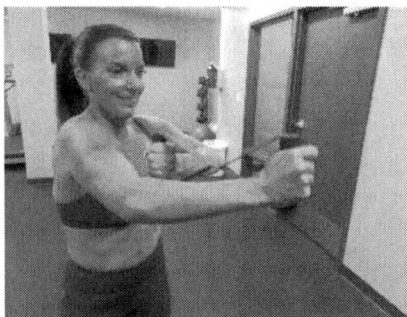

Aim to perform an exercise breathing count of no less than 7 seconds, and for no longer than 10 seconds.

Shoulders - Side and Front Lateral Superset

Iso-Bow® Side Lateral Raise – Left and Right Arm

Hold the Iso-Bow® slightly to one side with both hands, roughly half way between lap and shoulder level, keeping your elbows very slightly bent at all times.

Keeping the elbow of raised arm high in order to properly engage only the side deltoids, attempt to pull the Iso-Bow® down with your lower arm, and engage the side shoulder muscles, or deltoids, of the higher arm as you do so.

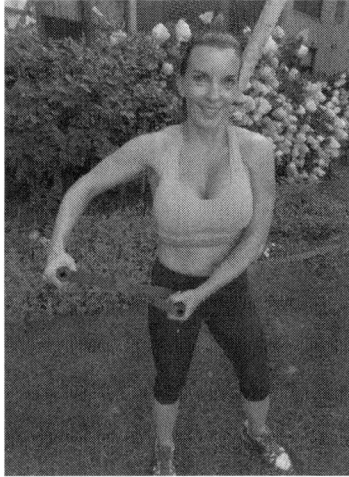

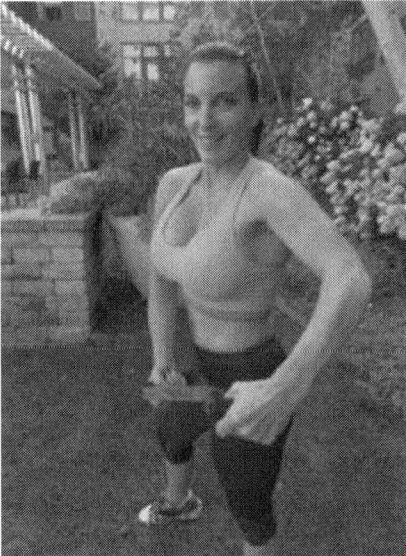

Breathe naturally and deeply in and out for about 10 full breaths, which will take about 1 second per breath.

Aim to perform an exercise breathing count of no less than 7 seconds, and for no longer than 10 seconds. Then repeat the exercise on the other side by reversing the hand and arm positions.

Iso-Bow® Front Raise – Left and Right Arm

Hold each handle of the Iso-Bow® firmly in front of you as shown. Keeping your leading elbow slightly bent, and use the front shoulder muscles to resist the downwards pull of the lower hand and arm.

Breathe naturally and deeply in and out for about 10 full breaths, which will take about 1 second per breath.

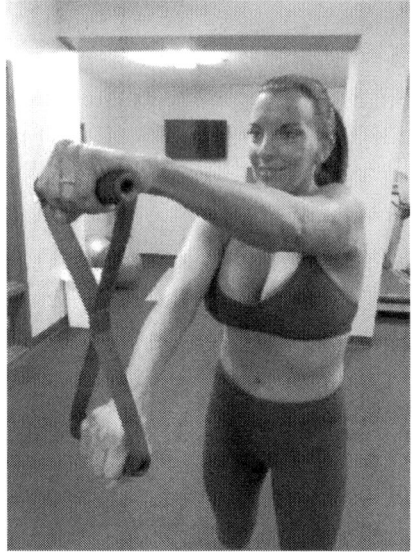

Aim to perform an exercise breathing count of no less than 7 seconds, and for no longer than 10 seconds.

Repeat the exercise on the other side by reversing the hand and arm positions.

Arms- Triceps and Biceps Superset

Iso-Bow® Triceps Press Down Over Knee

Put one foot on a solid object such as bench or a chair, and place the Iso-Bow® in a comfortable position face downwards, close to the knee and hold both handles.

Bend the arms and learn forwards over the knee, and keeping your elbows close to your body at all times while pushing down on each handle to engage the triceps muscles of both arms as you attempt to push your body back into an upright position.

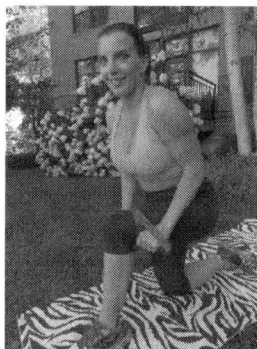

You won't be able to move, because your bodyweight and your upper body muscles will prevent you.

Breathe naturally and deeply in and out for about 10 full breaths, which will take about 1 second per breath.

Aim to perform an exercise breathing count of no less than 7 seconds, and for no longer than 10 seconds.

Dual Iso-Bow® Foot Loop Biceps Curl

Lean against a solid object, or sit on a chair, car seat or bench, and place the looped ends of two Iso-Bows® around one foot.

Raise that leg slightly until you assume the arm curl position, and then use your leg to provide opposing immovable resistance for your biceps muscles.

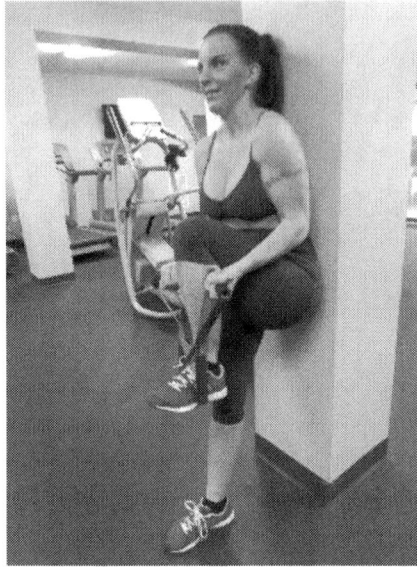

Breathe naturally and deeply in and out for about 10 full breaths, which will take about 1 second per breath.

Aim to perform an exercise breathing count of no less than 7 seconds, and for no longer than 10 seconds.

Lower Back and Abdominals Superset

Iso-Bow® Superhero Trunk and Leg Raise

Lying face down on the ground, grip the Iso-Bow® with both hands above your head. Lift your chest and legs slightly off the floor to engage the back, glutes, hamstrings and core muscles, with the Iso-Bow® to help stabilize you.

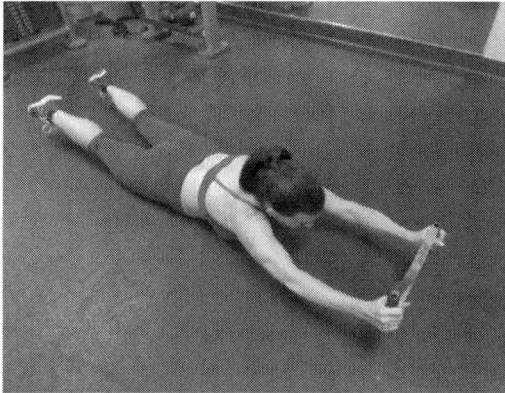

Breathe naturally and deeply in and out for about 10 full breaths, which will take about 1 second per breath.

Aim to perform an exercise breathing count of no less than 7 seconds, and for no longer than 10 seconds.

Iso-Bow® V-Sit Side to Side

Lay down, and
raise your legs
and torso off the
floor by curling
the spine,
gripping the Iso-
Bow® securely
with both hands
close to your mid-
section.

Twist the Iso-Bow® to one side as you engage the abdominal and oblique muscles.

Breathe naturally and deeply in and out for about 10 full breaths, which will take about 1 second per breath.

Aim to perform an exercise breathing count of no less than

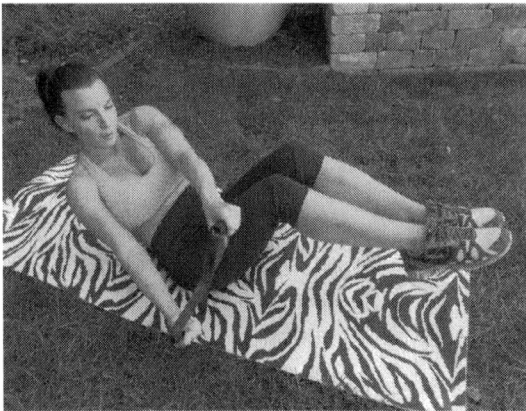

7 seconds, and for no longer than 10 seconds. Repeat the exercise on the other side of your body.

The ISO90™ Course Week 7 at a Glance

Legs – Quadriceps and Hamstring Superset

- △ *Iso-Bow® Leg Extension – Single Leg - Left and Right Leg*
- △ *Iso-Bow® Hamstring Seated Curl – Left and Right Leg*

Calf's

- △ *Calf Single Leg Wall Push – Left and Right Leg*

Upper Back and Chest Superset

- △ *Iso-Bow® Upper Back Seated Knee Brace Row*
- △ *Iso-Bow® Chest Press and Upper Back Row - Left and Right*

Shoulders - Side and Front Lateral Superset

- △ *Iso-Bow® Side Lateral Raise – Left and Right Arm*
- △ *Iso-Bow® Front Raise – Left and Right Arm*

Arms- Triceps and Biceps Superset

- △ *Iso-Bow® Triceps Press Down Over Knee*
- △ *Dual Iso-Bow® Foot Loop Biceps Curl*

Lower Back and Abdominals Superset

- △ *Iso-Bow® Superhero Trunk and Leg Raise*
- △ *Iso-Bow® V-Sit Side to Side*

The ISO90™ Course Week 8

Week 8 Notes

△ Continue to try to slightly increase the intensity used with all exercises, and to slightly reduce the amount of rest time between exercises.

△ Apply approximately 75% of your maximum potential intensity to each exercise.

Perform only one 7 second isometric exercise contraction. *(Don't start counting until you've fully applied the desired level of intensity)*

△ Before you begin the full isometric contraction part of the exercise, take between 2 and 3 additional seconds to perform Dynamic Flexation™ to help you properly engage the muscles and joints. Similarly, at the end of each isometric exercise, do the same in reverse as you disengage from the exercise over a period of between 2 and 3 seconds.

△ Perform the workout EVERY DAY, Monday to Friday inclusive, and take Saturday and Sunday as rest days over the weekend.

△ NEW Technique – Supersets. 2 exercises linked together, each for opposing muscle groups. Take no rest between each of these exercises. More information is in the superset section on page 29.

△ 5 NEW Exercises.

Legs – Quadriceps and Hamstring Supersets

Iso-Bow® Leg Extension – Single Leg - Left and Right

Sit on a chair, car seat or bench, raise one knee and place the Iso-Bow® comfortably around the lower part of your leg, close to your foot.

Hold the handles firmly, keep your back straight, bending only from the hips, and lean back slightly as you try to raise your leg and push it forwards, keeping your toes upwards at all times.

Breathe naturally and deeply in and out for about 10 full breaths, which will take about 1 second per breath.

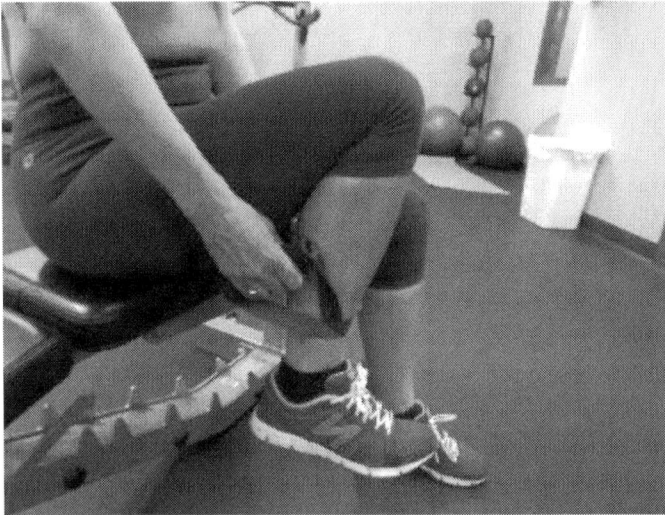

Aim to perform an exercise breathing count of no less than 7 seconds, and for no longer than 10 seconds. Switch legs and repeat the exercise with the other leg.

Iso-Bow® Hamstring Seated Curl – Left and Right Leg

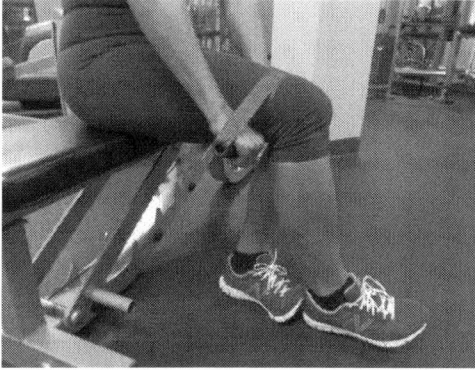

Sit on a chair, car seat or bench, and push the Iso-Bow® comfortably down over one leg to help prevent it from raising up during the exercise.

Place one foot directly in front of the other, so the heel of the leading foot is touching the toes of your rear foot, and turn up the toes to create a firmer connection.

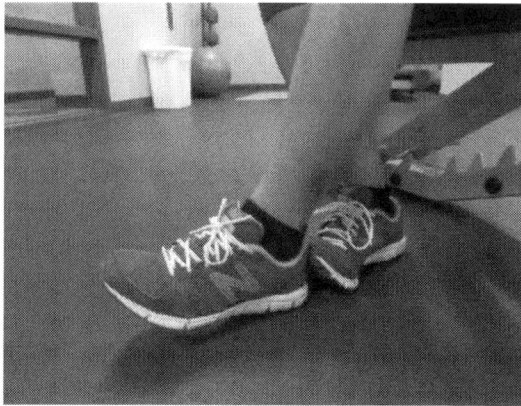

Try to draw back the leading foot by engaging the hamstring muscles of the rear upper thigh.

Breathe naturally and deeply in and out for about 10 full breaths, which will take about 1 second per breath.

Aim to perform an exercise breathing count of no less than 7 seconds, and for no longer than 10 seconds. Repeat the exercise for the other leg, by swapping the leg and foot positions.

NEW - Dual Iso-Bow® Stirrup Squat

Place the looped handle side of each Iso-Bow®
around each
foot as shown.
Bend your
knees deeply to
assume the
squat position,
bending your
torso only at
the hips, and
keeping your back straight and upright at all times.

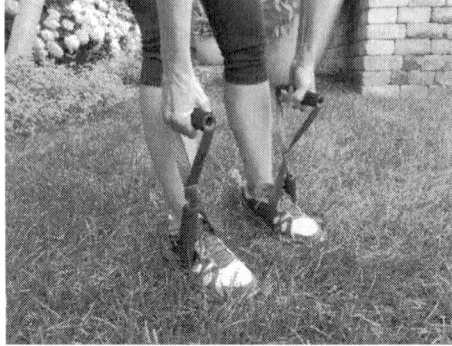

Grip each Iso-Bow® handle firmly, and attempt to
stand up straight by engaging your upper thigh and glute
muscles. Naturally
you won't be able to
move, but continue
your attempt to
stand up, while
maintain the perfect
mid-squat position as
you do so.

Breathe naturally
and deeply in and
out for about 10 full
breaths, which will
take about 1 second
per breath.

Aim to perform an exercise breathing count of no
less than 7 seconds, and for no longer than 10 seconds.

NEW - Standing Hamstring Wall Curl – Left and Right Leg

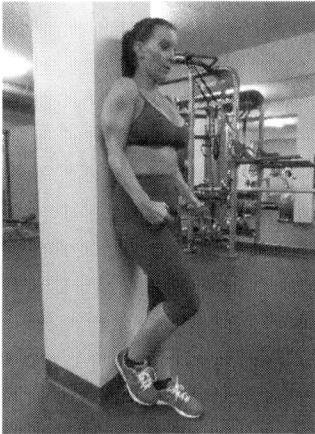

Stand with your back against a solid wall, or door which you can press your foot against. If you're using a vehicle you can use the wheel and tyre ('tire' in American vernacular) as a foot engagement point.

Bend one knee and place the heel of that leg against the wall, door, or vehicle to engage the hamstring muscles. Attempt to raise the heel as you press against the immovable object, and stabilize yourself with the other

leg positioned slightly forwards to help you push backwards, and with an Iso-Bow® in front of you.

Breathe naturally and deeply in and out for about 10 full breaths, which will take about 1 second per breath. Aim to perform an exercise breathing count of no less than 7 seconds, and for no longer than 10 seconds. Repeat the exercise for the other leg, by swapping the leg and foot positions.

Calf's

Calf Single Leg Wall Push – Left and Right Leg

Hold an Iso-Bow® for balance, and place it together with your hands against a wall, a car, a door frame, or any other solid object which is immovable by human muscle power alone.

With one leg behind you in a firm position, and with the ball of your foot on the floor, raise the heel slightly as you engage your calf muscles, pushing against the immovable object.

Breathe naturally and deeply in and out for about 10 full breaths, which will take about 1 second per breath.

Aim to perform an exercise breathing count of no less than 7 seconds, and for no longer than 10 seconds.

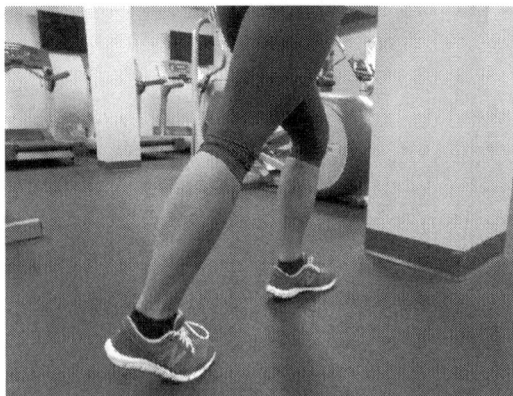

Switch legs and repeat the exercise with the other leg.

Upper Back and Chest Supersets

Iso-Bow® Upper Back Seated Knee Brace Row

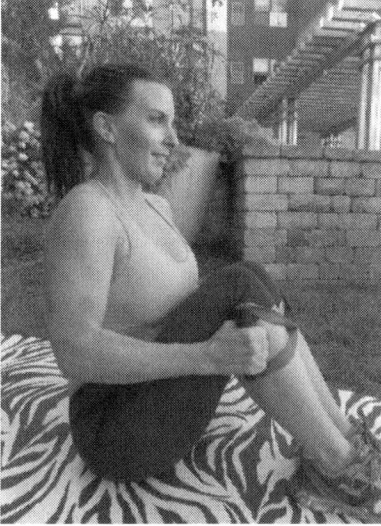

Sit upright on the floor with your feet under a secure object that won't tip over, bending forwards only from the hips, and keeping your back straight at all times.

Wrap the Iso-Bow® comfortably around both knees, and pull back with each handle to engage your upper back muscles, keeping your

elbows close to your body as you do so.

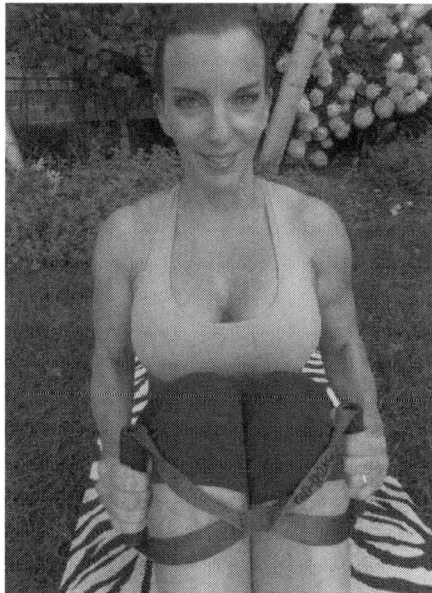

Breathe naturally and deeply in and out for about 10 full breaths, which will take about 1 second per breath.

Aim to perform an exercise breathing count of no less than 7 seconds, and for no longer than 10 seconds.

156

Iso-Bow® Chest Press and Upper Back Row – Left and Right

With one arm in front of you roughly parallel to the

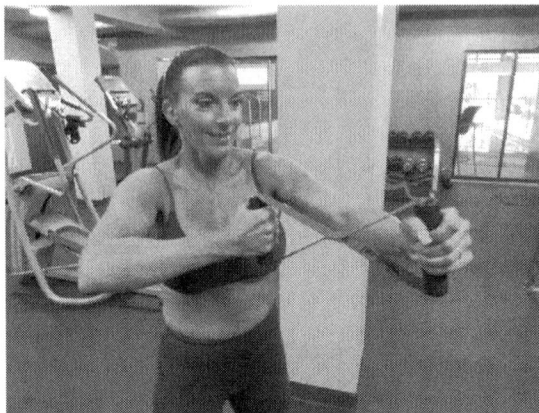

floor, push one end of the Iso-Bow® forwards, and at the same time pull the other handle backwards,

keep the elbows of both arms slightly bent at all times.

Breathe naturally and deeply in and out for about 10 full breaths, which will take about 1 second per breath.

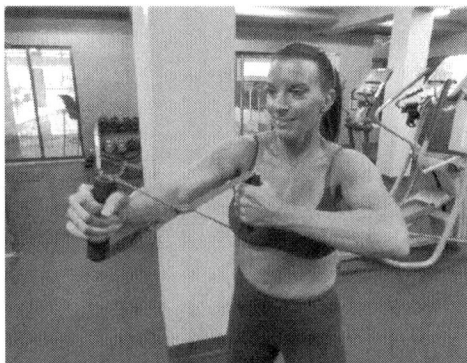

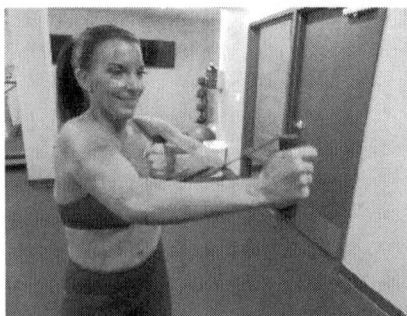

Aim to perform an exercise breathing count of no less than 7 seconds, and for no longer than 10 seconds.

NEW - Iso-Bow® Latissimus Overhead Pull Apart

Grip the Iso-Bow® handle, placing the central section comfortably and flat, just above the top of the head. In this position, try to pull your hands apart, engaging the latissimus muscles of the upper back as you do so.

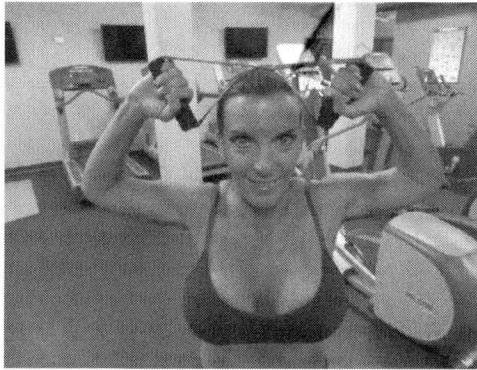

Breathe naturally and deeply in and out for about 10 full breaths, which will take about 1 second per breath. Aim to perform an exercise breathing count of no less than 7 seconds, and for no longer than 10 seconds.

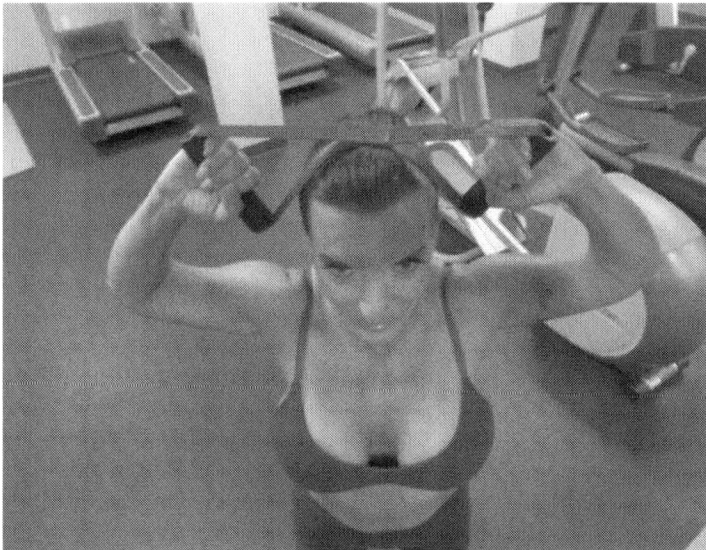

NEW - Iso-Bow® Cradle Cross Press

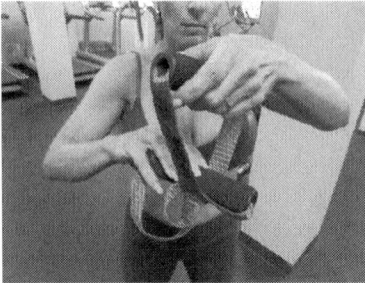

Cradle the Iso-Bow® to make a shorter hand grip, cross it in front of you at chest level, with your arms roughly parallel to the floor, and push in opposing directions sideways to engage your chest muscles.

Breathe naturally and deeply in and out for about 10 full breaths, which will take about 1 second per breath. Aim to perform an exercise breathing count of no less than 7 seconds, and for no longer than 10 seconds.

Shoulders - Side and Front Lateral Superset

Iso-Bow® Side Lateral Raise – Left and Right Arm

Hold the Iso-Bow® slightly to one side with both hands, roughly half way between lap and shoulder level, keeping your elbows very slightly bent at all times.

Keeping the elbow of raised arm high in order to properly engage only the side deltoids, attempt to pull the Iso-Bow® down with your lower arm, and engage the side shoulder muscles, or deltoids, of the higher arm as you do so.

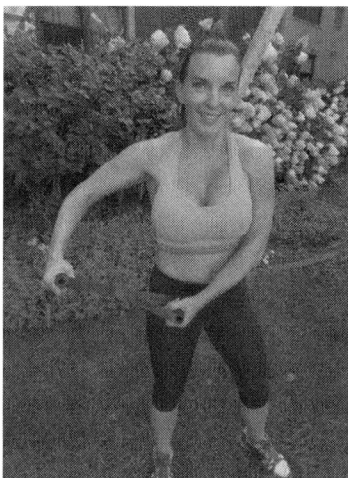

Breathe naturally and deeply in and out for about 10 full breaths, which will take about 1 second per breath.

Aim to perform an exercise breathing count of no less than 7 seconds, and for no longer than 10 seconds. Then repeat the exercise on the other side by reversing the hand and arm positions.

160

Iso-Bow® Front Raise – Left and Right Arm

Hold each handle of the Iso-Bow® firmly in front of you as shown. Keeping your leading elbow slightly bent, and use the front shoulder muscles to resist the downwards pull of the lower hand and arm.

Breathe naturally and deeply in and out for about 10 full breaths, which will take about 1 second per breath.

Aim to perform an exercise breathing count of no less than 7 seconds, and for no longer than 10 seconds.

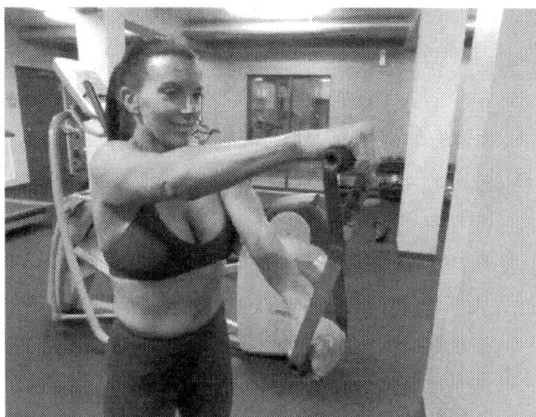

Repeat the exercise on the other side by reversing the hand and arm positions.

Arms- Triceps and Biceps Supersets

Iso-Bow® Triceps Press Down Over Knee

Put one foot on a solid object such as bench or a chair, and place the Iso-Bow® in a comfortable position face downwards, close to the knee and hold both handles.

Bend the arms and learn forwards over the knee, and keeping your elbows close to your body at all times while pushing down on each handle to engage the triceps muscles of both arms as you attempt to push your body back into an upright position.

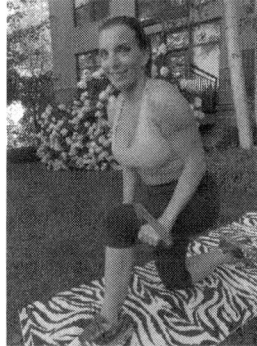

You won't be able to move, because your bodyweight and your upper body muscles will prevent you.

Breathe naturally and deeply in and out for about 10 full breaths, which will take about 1 second per breath.

Aim to perform an exercise breathing count of no less than 7 seconds, and for no longer than 10 seconds.

Dual Iso-Bow® Foot Loop Biceps Curl

Lean against a solid object, or sit on a chair, car seat or bench, and place the looped ends of two Iso-Bows® around one foot.

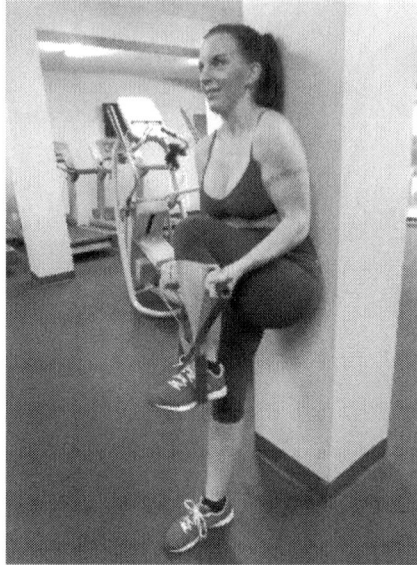

Raise that leg slightly until you assume the arm curl position, and then use your leg to provide opposing immovable resistance for your biceps muscles.

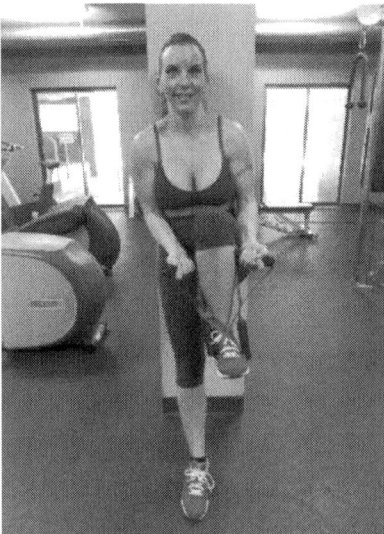

Breathe naturally and deeply in and out for about 10 full breaths, which will take about 1 second per breath.

Aim to perform an exercise breathing count of no less than 7 seconds, and for no longer than 10 seconds.

NEW - Iso-Bow® Biceps and Triceps Cradle Press-Curl (Left)

Firstly, you'll exercise the biceps of your right arm, and triceps muscles of your left arm.

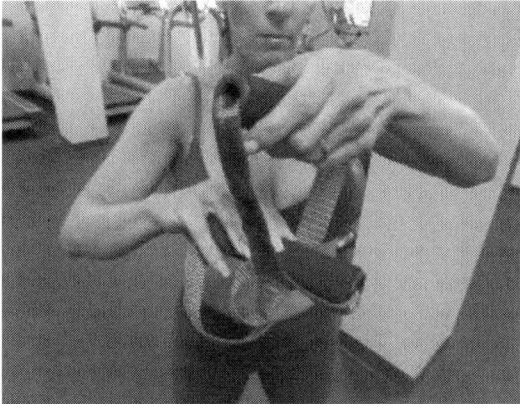

Cradle the Iso-Bow with your left hand, gripping the top with your right hand facing up. Grip the cradled side of the Iso-Bow with the left hand facing down.

Keep both elbows close to your body, and with your right arm across the front of you at waist height. In this position, press down with the left hand, and at the same time press up with the right, to engage both the Biceps and Triceps muscles simultaneously.

Breathe naturally and deeply in and out for about 10 full breaths, which will take about 1 second per breath.

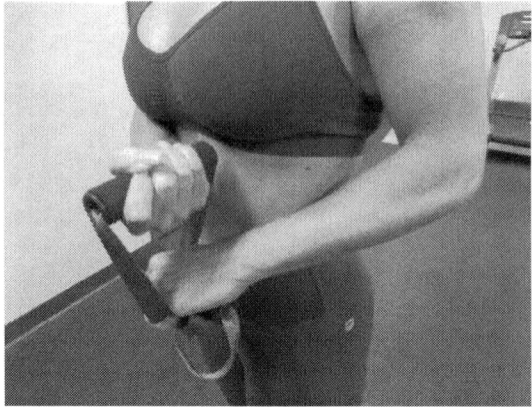

Aim to perform an exercise breathing count of no less than 7 seconds, and for no longer than 10 seconds.

Next, you'll need to perform the same exercise in reverse so that you now engage the biceps of your left arm, and triceps muscles of your right arm.

Iso-Bow® Biceps and Triceps Cradle Press-Curl (Right Side)

Cradle the Iso-Bow® with your right hand, gripping the top with your left hand facing up. Grip the cradled side of the Iso-Bow with the right hand facing down.

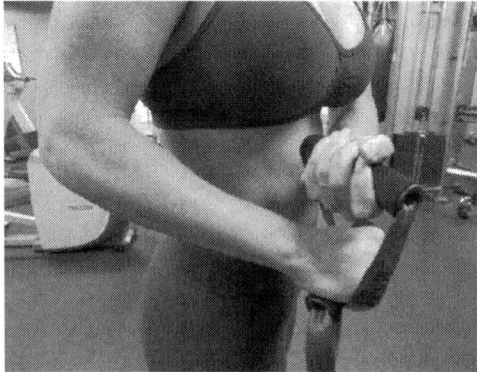

Keep both elbows close to your body, and with your left arm across the front of you at waist height. In this position, press down with the right hand, and at the same time press up with the

left, to engage both the Biceps and Triceps muscles simultaneously.

Breathe naturally and deeply in and out for about 10 full breaths, which will take about 1 second per breath.

Aim to perform an exercise breathing count of no less than 7 seconds, and for no longer than 10 seconds.

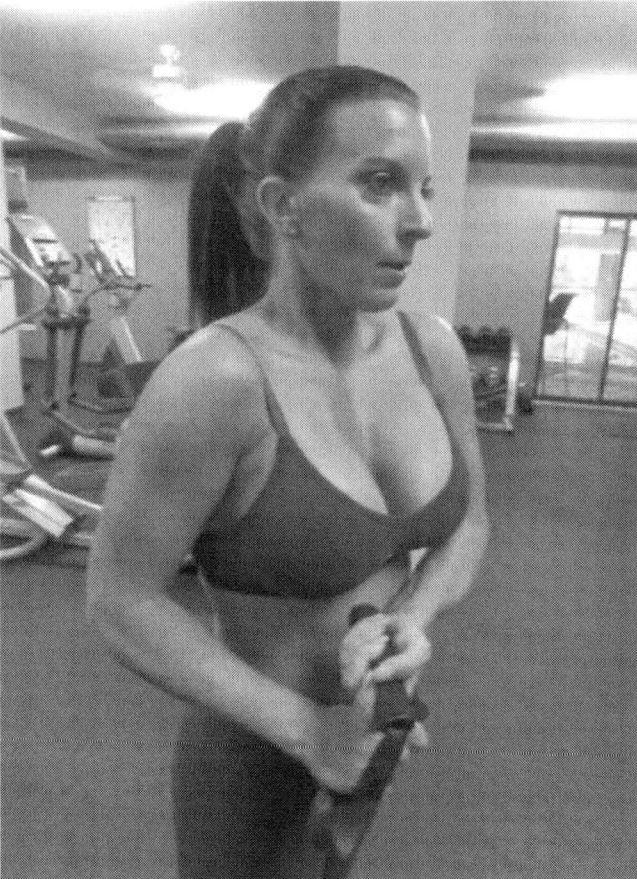

Lower Back and Abdominals Supersets

Iso-Bow® Superhero Trunk and Leg Raise

Lying face down on the ground, grip the Iso-Bow®
with both hands above your head. Lift your chest and legs slightly off the floor to engage the back,

glutes, hamstrings and core muscles, with the Iso-Bow® to help stabilize you.

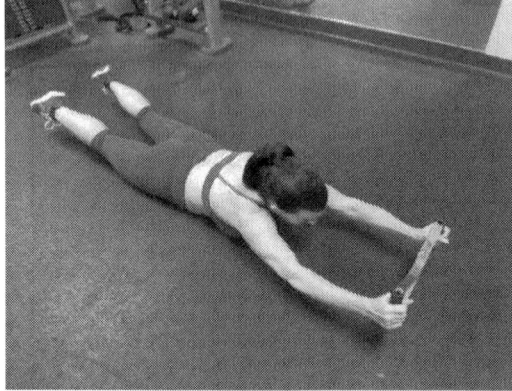

Breathe naturally and deeply in and out for about 10 full breaths, which will take about 1 second per breath.

Aim to perform an exercise breathing count of no less than 7 seconds, and for no longer than 10 seconds.

Iso-Bow® V-Sit Side to Side

Lay down, and raise your legs and torso off the floor by curling the spine, gripping the Iso-Bow® securely with both hands close to your mid-section.

Twist the Iso-Bow® to one side as you engage the abdominal and oblique muscles.

Breathe naturally and deeply in and out for about 10 full breaths, which will take about 1 second per breath.

Aim to perform an exercise breathing count of no less than

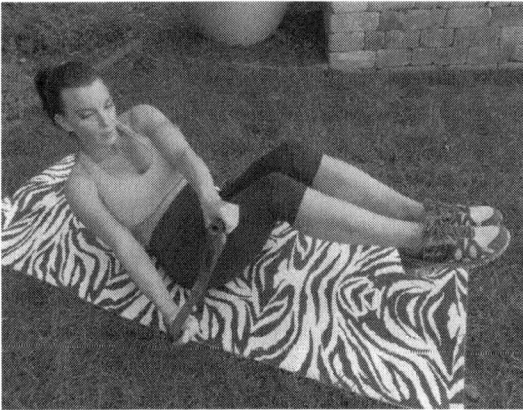

7 seconds, and for no longer than 10 seconds. Repeat the exercise on the other side of your body.

The ISO90™ Course Week 8 at a Glance

Legs – Quadriceps and Hamstring Supersets

- △ *Iso-Bow® Leg Extension – Single Leg - Left and Right*
- △ *Iso-Bow® Hamstring Seated Curl – Left and Right Leg*
- △ *NEW - Dual Iso-Bow® Stirrup Squat*
- △ *NEW - Standing Hamstring Wall Curl – Left and Right Leg*

Calf's

- △ *Calf Single Leg Wall Push – Left and Right Leg*

Upper Back and Chest Supersets

- △ *Iso-Bow® Upper Back Seated Knee Brace Row*
- △ *Iso-Bow® Chest Press and Upper Back Row – Left and Right*
- △ *NEW - Iso-Bow® Latissimus Overhead Pull Apart*
- △ *NEW - Iso-Bow® Cradle Cross Press*

Shoulders - Side and Front Lateral Superset

- △ *Iso-Bow® Side Lateral Raise – Left and Right Arm*
- △ *Iso-Bow® Front Raise – Left and Right Arm*

Arms- Triceps and Biceps Supersets

- △ *Iso-Bow® Triceps Press Down Over Knee*
- △ *Dual Iso-Bow® Foot Loop Biceps Curl*
- △ *NEW - Iso-Bow® Biceps and Triceps Cradle Press-Curl (Left Side)*
- △ *Iso-Bow® Biceps and Triceps Cradle Press-Curl (Right Side)*

Lower Back and Abdominals Supersets

- △ *Iso-Bow® Superhero Trunk and Leg Raise*
- △ *Iso-Bow® V-Sit Side to Side*

169

The ISO90™ Course Week 9

Week 9 Notes

⚠ This week, you slightly DECREASE the intensity, while still trying to slightly reduce the amount of rest time between exercises.

⚠ Apply approximately 65% of your maximum potential intensity to each exercise.

Perform only one 7 second isometric exercise contraction. *(Don't start counting until you've fully applied the desired level of intensity)*

⚠ Before you begin the full isometric contraction part of the exercise, take between 2 and 3 additional seconds to perform Dynamic Flexation™ to help you properly engage the muscles and joints. Similarly, at the end of each isometric exercise, do the same in reverse as you disengage from the exercise over a period of between 2 and 3 seconds.

⚠ Perform the workout EVERY DAY with NO rest days.

⚠ NEW Technique – Supersets. 2 exercises linked together, each for opposing muscle groups. Take no rest between each of these exercises. More information is in the superset section on page 29.

⚠ 2 NEW Exercises.

Legs – Quadriceps and Hamstring Supersets

Iso-Bow® Leg Extension – Single Leg - Left and Right

Sit on a chair, car seat or bench, raise one knee and place the Iso-Bow® comfortably around the lower part of your leg, close to your foot.

Hold the handles firmly, keep your back straight, bending only from the hips, and lean back slightly as you try to raise your leg and push it forwards, keeping your toes upwards at all times.

Breathe naturally and deeply in and out for about 10 full breaths, which will take about 1 second per breath.

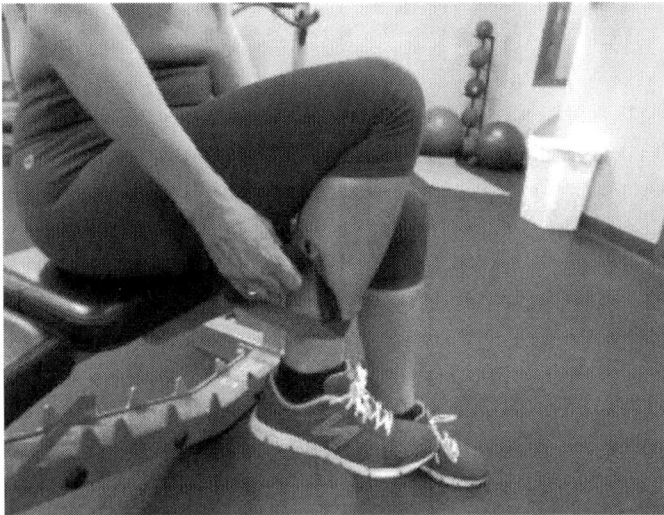

Aim to perform an exercise breathing count of no less than 7 seconds, and for no longer than 10 seconds. Switch legs and repeat the exercise with the other leg.

Iso-Bow® Hamstring Seated Curl – Left and Right Leg

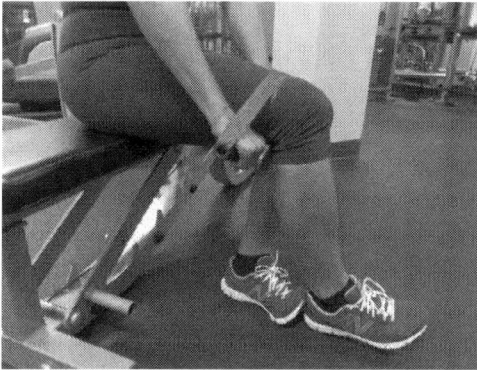

Sit on a chair, car seat or bench, and push the Iso-Bow® comfortably down over one leg to help prevent it from raising up during the exercise.

Place one foot directly in front of the other, so the heel of the leading foot is touching the toes of your rear foot, and turn up the toes to create a firmer connection.

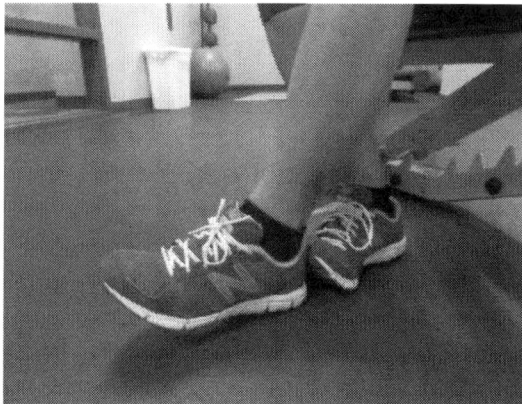

Try to draw back the leading foot by engaging the hamstring muscles of the rear upper thigh.

Breathe naturally and deeply in and out for about 10 full breaths, which will take about 1 second per breath.

Aim to perform an exercise breathing count of no less than 7 seconds, and for no longer than 10 seconds. Repeat the exercise for the other leg, by swapping the leg and foot positions.

Dual Iso-Bow® Stirrup Squat

Place the looped handle side of each Iso-Bow® around each foot as shown. Bend your knees deeply to assume the squat position, bending your torso only at the hips, and keeping your back straight and upright at all times.

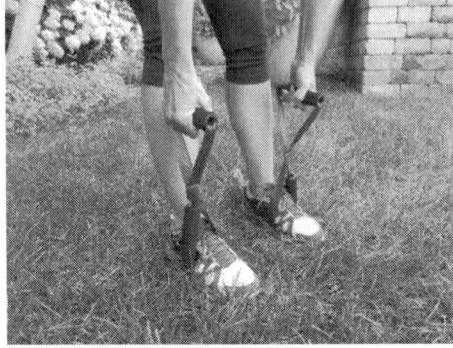

Grip each Iso-Bow® handle firmly, and attempt to stand up straight by engaging your upper thigh and glute muscles. Naturally you won't be able to move, but continue your attempt to stand up, while maintain the perfect mid-squat position as you do so.

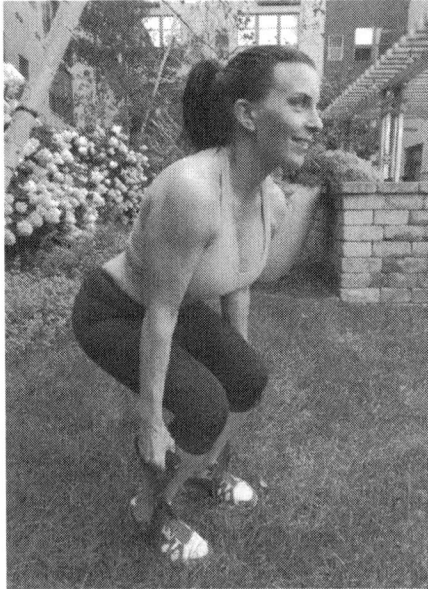

Breathe naturally and deeply in and out for about 10 full breaths, which will take about 1 second per breath.

Aim to perform an exercise breathing count of no less than 7 seconds, and for no longer than 10 seconds.

Standing Hamstring Wall Curl – Left and Right Leg

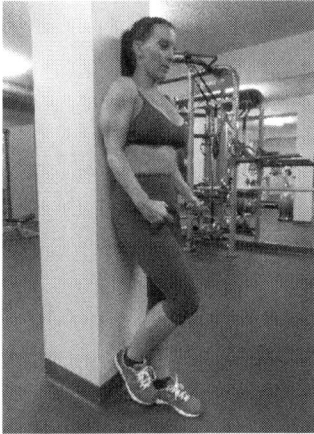

Stand with your back against a solid wall, or door which you can press your foot against. If you're using a vehicle you can use the wheel and tyre ('tire' in American vernacular) as a foot engagement point.

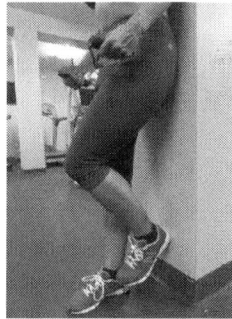

Bend one knee and place the heel of that leg against the wall, door, or vehicle to engage the hamstring muscles. Attempt to raise the heel as you press against the immovable object, and stabilize yourself with the other

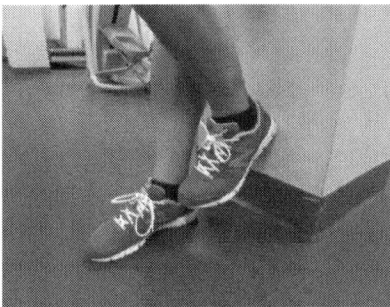

leg positioned slightly forwards to help you push backwards, and with an Iso-Bow® in front of you.

Breathe naturally and deeply in and out for about 10 full breaths, which will take about 1 second per breath. Aim to perform an exercise breathing count of no less than 7 seconds, and for no longer than 10 seconds. Repeat the exercise for the other leg, by swapping the leg and foot positions.

Calf's

Calf Single Leg Wall Push – Left and Right Leg

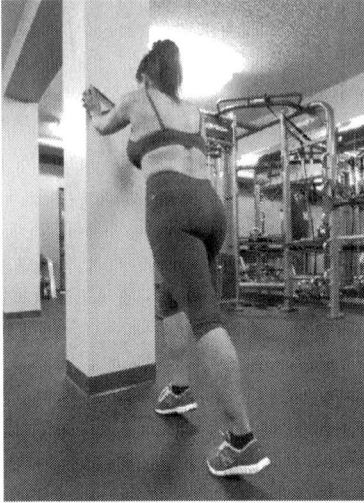

Hold an Iso-Bow® for balance, and place it together with your hands against a wall, a car, a door frame, or any other solid object which is immovable by human muscle power alone.

With one leg behind you in a firm position, and with the ball of your foot on the floor, raise the heel slightly as you engage your calf muscles, pushing against the immovable object.

Breathe naturally and deeply in and out for about 10 full breaths, which will take about 1 second per breath.

Aim to perform an exercise breathing count of no less than 7 seconds, and for no longer than 10 seconds.

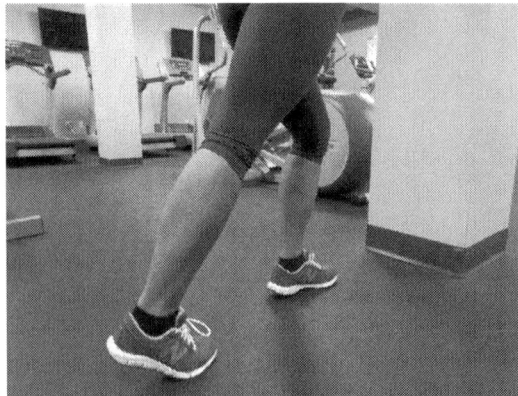

Switch legs and repeat the exercise with the other leg.

175

Upper Back and Chest Supersets

Iso-Bow® Upper Back Seated Knee Brace Row

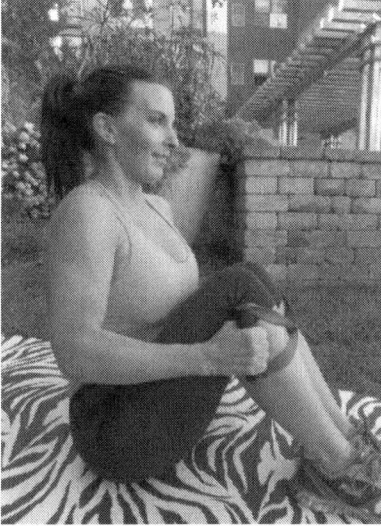

Sit upright on the floor with your feet under a secure object that won't tip over, bending forwards only from the hips, and keeping your back straight at all times.

Wrap the Iso-Bow® comfortably around both knees, and pull back with each handle to engage your upper back muscles, keeping your elbows close to your body as you do so.

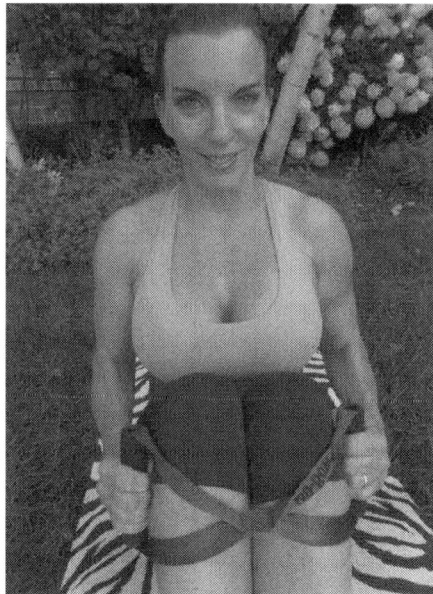

Breathe naturally and deeply in and out for about 10 full breaths, which will take about 1 second per breath.

Aim to perform an exercise breathing count of no less than 7 seconds, and for no longer than 10 seconds.

With one arm in front of you roughly parallel to the

floor, push one end of the Iso-Bow® forwards, and at the same time pull the other handle backwards, keep the elbows of both arms slightly bent at all times.

Breathe naturally and deeply in and out for about 10 full breaths, which will take about 1 second per breath.

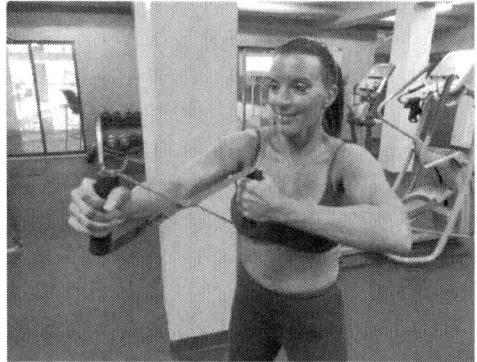

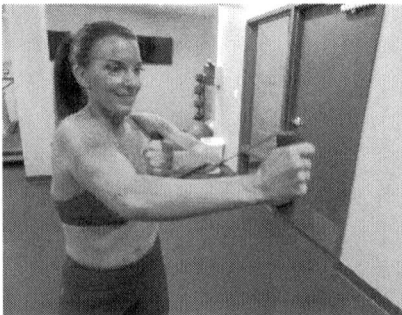

Aim to perform an exercise breathing count of no less than 7 seconds, and for no longer than 10 seconds.

Iso-Bow® Latissimus Overhead Pull Apart

Grip the Iso-Bow® handle, placing the central section comfortably and flat, just above the top of the head. In this position,

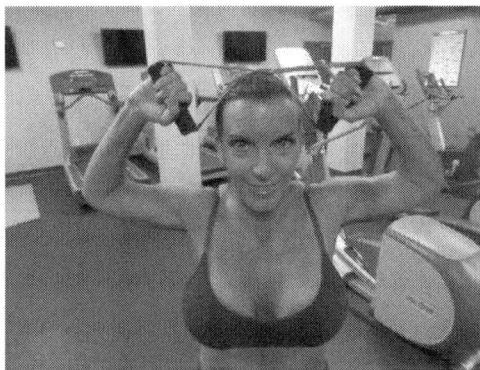

try to pull your hands apart, engaging the latissimus muscles of the upper back as you do so.

Breathe naturally and deeply in and out for about 10 full breaths, which will take about 1 second per breath. Aim to perform an exercise breathing count of no less than 7 seconds, and for no longer than 10 seconds.

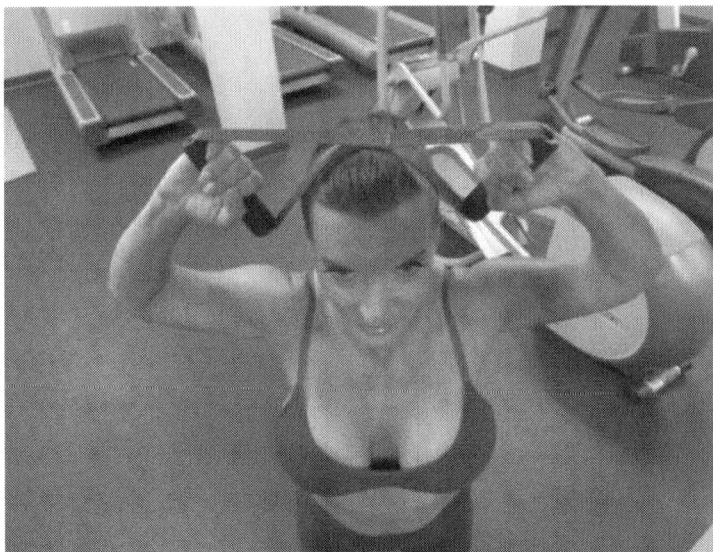

Iso-Bow® Cradle Cross Press

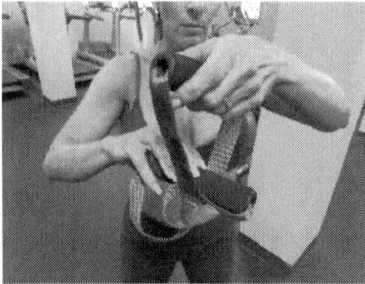

Cradle the Iso-Bow® to make a shorter hand grip, cross it in front of you at chest level, with your arms roughly parallel to the floor, and push in opposing directions sideways to engage your chest muscles.

Breathe naturally and deeply in and out for about 10 full breaths, which will take about 1 second per breath. Aim to perform an exercise breathing count of no less than 7 seconds, and for no longer than 10 seconds.

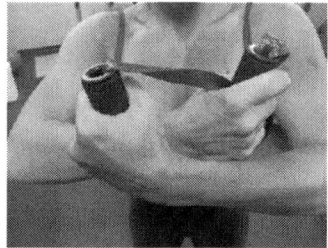

Shoulders - Side and Front Lateral Superset

Iso-Bow® Side Lateral Raise – Left and Right Arm

Hold the Iso-Bow® slightly to one side with both hands, roughly half way between lap and shoulder level, keeping your elbows very slightly bent at all times.

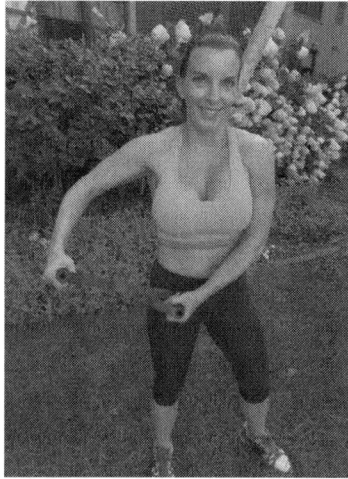

Keeping the elbow of raised arm high in order to properly engage only the side deltoids, attempt to pull the Iso-Bow® down with your lower arm, and engage the side shoulder muscles, or deltoids, of the higher arm as you do so.

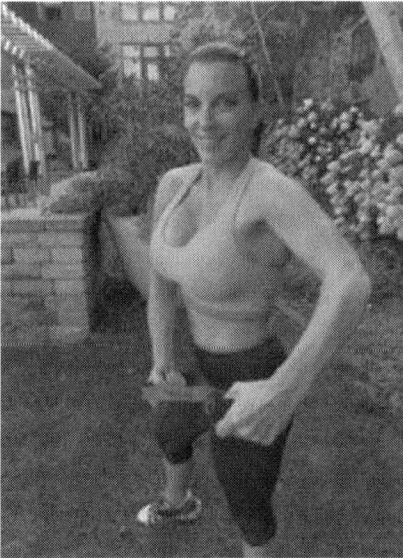

Breathe naturally and deeply in and out for about 10 full breaths, which will take about 1 second per breath.

Aim to perform an exercise breathing count of no less than 7 seconds, and for no longer than 10 seconds. Then repeat the exercise on the other side by reversing the hand and arm positions.

Iso-Bow® Front Raise – Left and Right Arm

Hold each handle of the Iso-Bow® firmly in front of you as shown. Keeping your leading elbow slightly bent, and use the front shoulder muscles to resist the downwards pull of the lower hand and arm.

Breathe naturally and deeply in and out for about 10 full breaths, which will take about 1 second per breath.

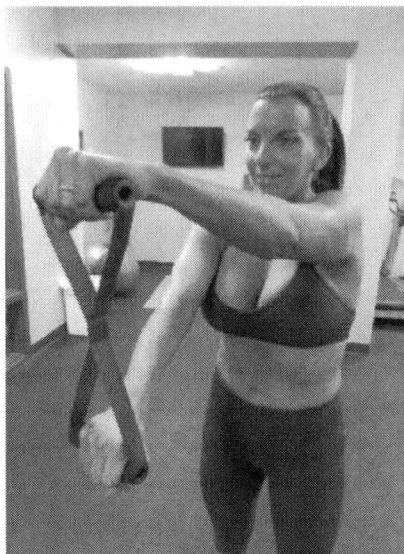

Aim to perform an exercise breathing count of no less than 7 seconds, and for no longer than 10 seconds.

Repeat the exercise on the other side by reversing the hand and arm positions.

Arms- Triceps and Biceps Supersets

Iso-Bow® Triceps Press Down Over Knee

Put one foot on a solid object such as bench or a chair, and place the Iso-Bow® in a comfortable position face downwards, close to the knee and hold both handles.

Bend the arms and learn forwards over the knee, and keeping your elbows close to your body at all times while pushing down on each handle to engage the triceps muscles of both arms as you attempt to push your body back into an upright position.

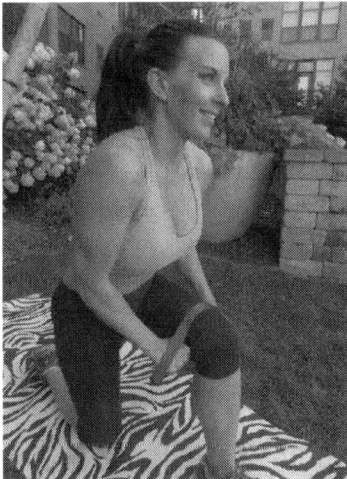

You won't be able to move, because your bodyweight and your upper body muscles will prevent you.

Breathe naturally and deeply in and out for about 10 full breaths, which will take about 1 second per breath.

Aim to perform an exercise breathing count of no less than 7 seconds, and for no longer than 10 seconds.

Dual Iso-Bow® Foot Loop Biceps Curl

Lean against a solid object, or sit on a chair, car seat or bench, and place the looped ends of two Iso-Bows® around one foot.

Raise that leg slightly until you assume the arm curl position, and then use your leg to provide opposing immovable resistance for your biceps muscles.

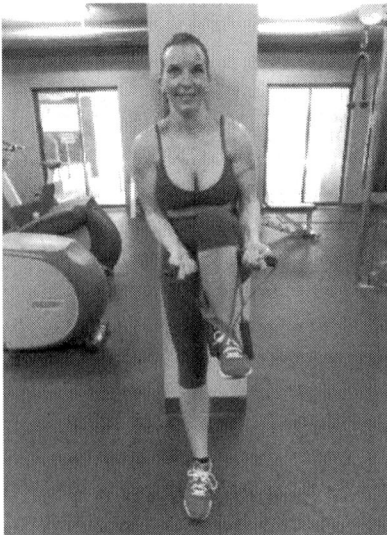

Breathe naturally and deeply in and out for about 10 full breaths, which will take about 1 second per breath.

Aim to perform an exercise breathing count of no less than 7 seconds, and for no longer than 10 seconds.

Iso-Bow® Biceps and Triceps Cradle Press-Curl (Left Side)

Firstly, you'll exercise the biceps of your right arm, and triceps muscles of your left arm.

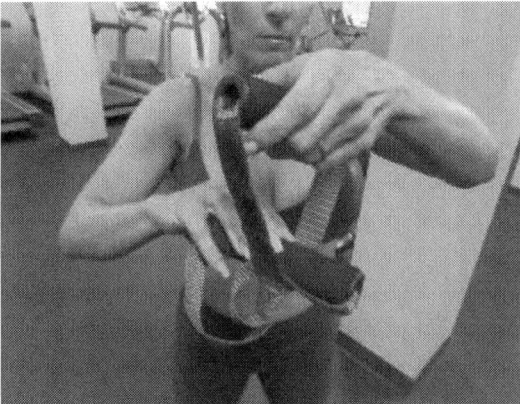

Cradle the Iso-Bow with your left hand, gripping the top with your right hand facing up. Grip the cradled side of the Iso-Bow with the left hand facing down.

Keep both elbows close to your body, and with your right arm across the front of you at waist height. In this position, press down with the left hand, and at the same time press up with the right, to engage both the Biceps and Triceps muscles simultaneously.

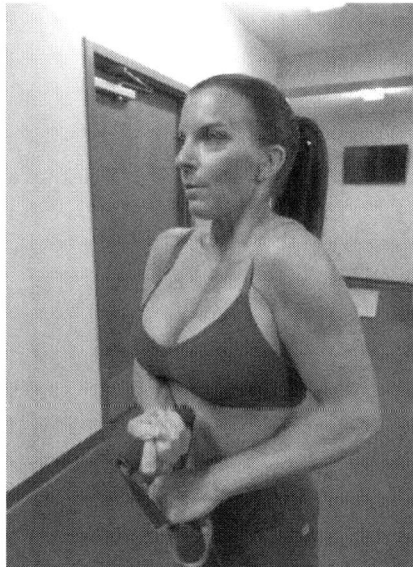

184

Breathe naturally and deeply in and out for about 10 full breaths, which will take about 1 second per breath.

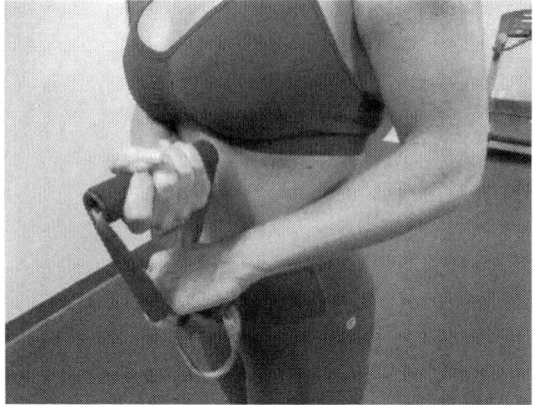

Aim to perform an exercise breathing count of no less than 7 seconds, and for no longer than 10 seconds.

Next, you'll need to perform the same exercise in reverse so that you now engage the biceps of your left arm, and triceps muscles of your right arm.

Iso-Bow® Biceps and Triceps Cradle Press-Curl (Right Side)

Cradle the Iso-Bow® with your right hand, gripping the top with your left hand facing up. Grip the cradled side of the Iso-Bow with the right hand facing down.

Keep both elbows close to your body, and with your left arm across the front of you at waist height. In this position, press down with the right hand, and at the same time press up with the

left, to engage both the Biceps and Triceps muscles simultaneously.

Breathe naturally and deeply in and out for about 10 full breaths, which will take about 1 second per breath.

Aim to perform an exercise breathing count of no less than 7 seconds, and for no longer than 10 seconds.

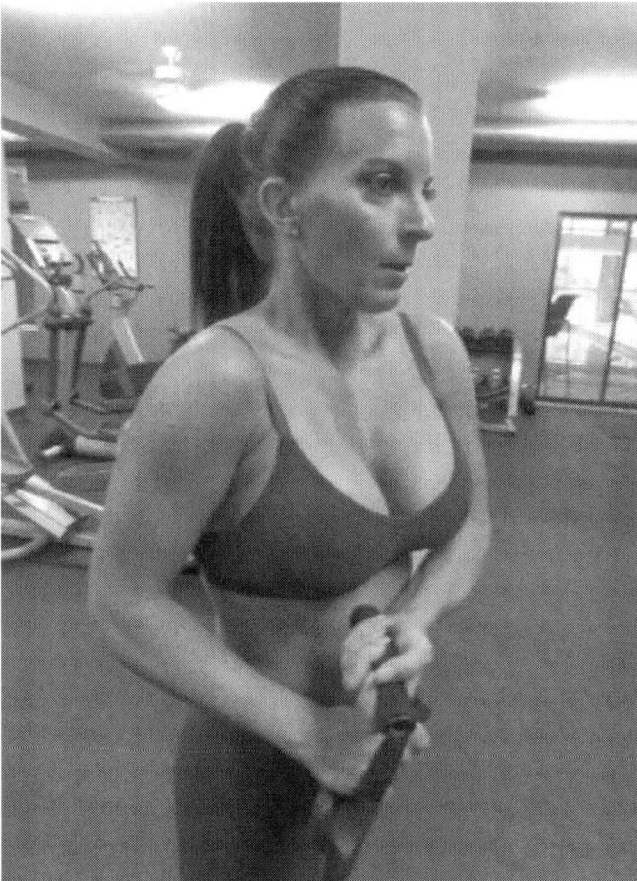

Lower Back and Abdominals Supersets

Iso-Bow® Superhero Trunk and Leg Raise

Lying face down on the ground, grip the Iso-Bow® with both hands above your head. Lift your chest and legs slightly off the floor to engage the back, glutes, hamstrings and core muscles, with the Iso-Bow® to help stabilize you.

Breathe naturally and deeply in and out for about 10 full breaths, which will take about 1 second per breath.

Aim to perform an exercise breathing count of no less than 7 seconds, and for no longer than 10 seconds.

Iso-Bow® V-Sit Side to Side

Lay down, and raise your legs and torso off the floor by curling the spine, gripping the Iso-Bow® securely with both hands close to your mid-section.

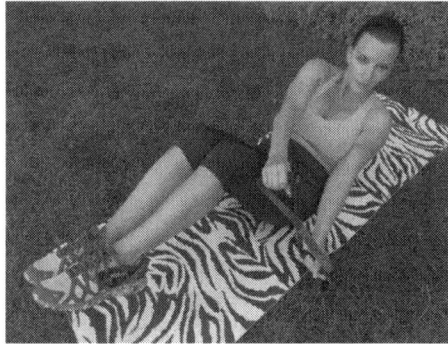

Twist the Iso-Bow® to one side as you engage the abdominal and oblique muscles.

Breathe naturally and deeply in and out for about 10 full breaths, which will take about 1 second per breath.

Aim to perform an exercise breathing count of no less than 7 seconds, and for no longer than 10 seconds. Repeat the exercise on the other side of your body.

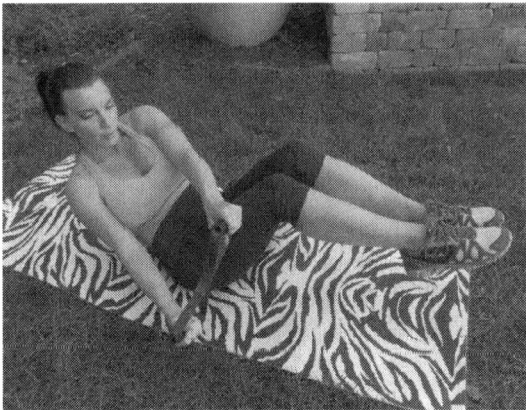

NEW - Dual Iso-Bow® Bent Leg Deadlift

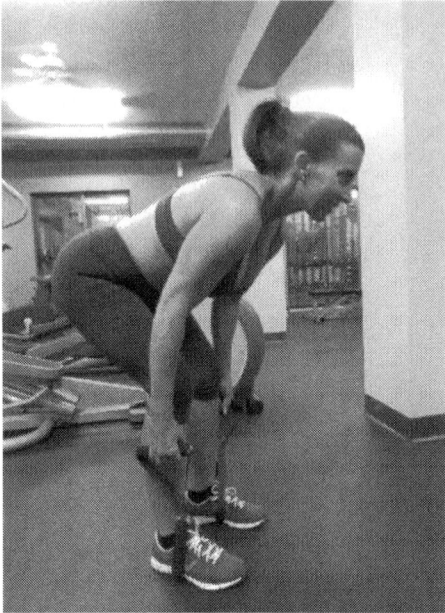

Place the loop handle of both Iso-Bows® around each foot as shown. Hold each handle firmly while maintaining a perfect bent-knee, semi squat position with your back straight at all times, then attempt to slowly stand up straight.

Engage the muscles of the glutes, hamstrings, lower back, thighs, and other core muscles, while the Iso-Bows® secured by your feet prevent any movement from taking place.

Breathe naturally and deeply in and out for about 10 full breaths, which will take about 1 second per breath.

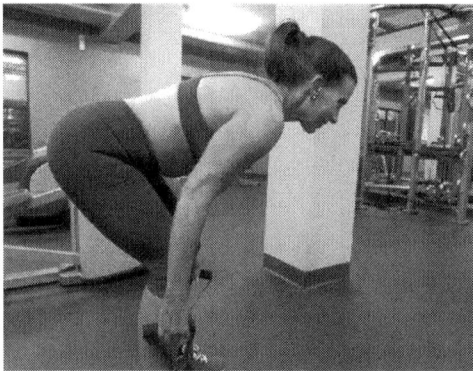

Aim to perform an exercise breathing count of no less than 7 seconds, and for no longer than 10 seconds.

NEW - Iso-Bow® Standing Knee Raise

Stand upright and raise one knee in front of you, with the Iso-Bow® facing downwards to cover it. Maintain your balance at all times by engaging your core muscles, and don't worry if this takes a little practice before you can do it perfectly.

Repeat the exercise with the other leg. Then, slightly curl your body forwards and downwards by contracting the abdominals, at the same time, attempt to raise the knee resisted by the Iso-Bow®.

Breathe deeply and naturally for about 10 full breaths, at a rate of about 1 second per breath. Aim to perform the breathing exercise count of no less than 7 seconds, and for no longer than 10 seconds.

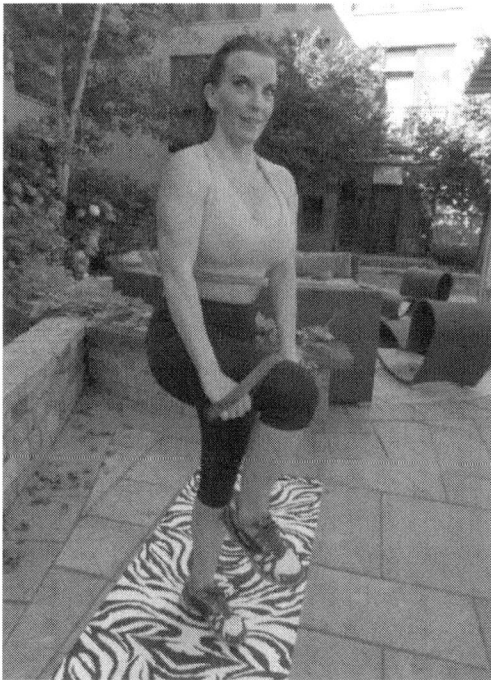

190

The ISO90™ Course Week 9 at a Glance

Legs – Quadriceps and Hamstring Supersets

- Iso-Bow® Leg Extension – Single Leg - Left and Right
- Iso-Bow® Hamstring Seated Curl – Left and Right Leg
- Dual Iso-Bow® Stirrup Squat
- Standing Hamstring Wall Curl – Left and Right Leg

Calf's

- Calf Single Leg Wall Push – Left and Right Leg

Upper Back and Chest Supersets

- Iso-Bow® Upper Back Seated Knee Brace Row
- Iso-Bow® Chest Press and Upper Back Row – Left and Right
- Iso-Bow® Latissimus Overhead Pull Apart
- Iso-Bow® Cradle Cross Press

Shoulders - Side and Front Lateral Superset

- Iso-Bow® Side Lateral Raise – Left and Right Arm
- Iso-Bow® Front Raise – Left and Right Arm

Arms- Triceps and Biceps Supersets

- Iso-Bow® Triceps Press Down Over Knee
- Dual Iso-Bow® Foot Loop Biceps Curl
- Iso-Bow® Biceps and Triceps Cradle Press-Curl (Left Side)
- Iso-Bow® Biceps and Triceps Cradle Press-Curl (Right Side)

Lower Back and Abdominals Supersets

- Iso-Bow® Superhero Trunk and Leg Raise
- Iso-Bow® V-Sit Side to Side
- NEW - Dual Iso-Bow® Bent Leg Deadlift
- NEW - Iso-Bow® Standing Knee Raise

The ISO90™ Course Week 10

Week 10 Notes

△ Increase the intensity used with all exercises, and as always, try to slightly reduce the amount of rest time between exercises.

△ Apply approximately 70% of your maximum potential intensity to each exercise.

Perform only one 7 second isometric exercise contraction. *(Don't start counting until you've fully applied the desired level of intensity)*

△ Before you begin the full isometric contraction part of the exercise, take between 2 and 3 additional seconds to perform Dynamic Flexation™ to help you properly engage the muscles and joints. Similarly, at the end of each isometric exercise, do the same in reverse as you disengage from the exercise over a period of between 2 and 3 seconds.

△ Perform the workout EVERY DAY with NO rest days.

△ New Routine.

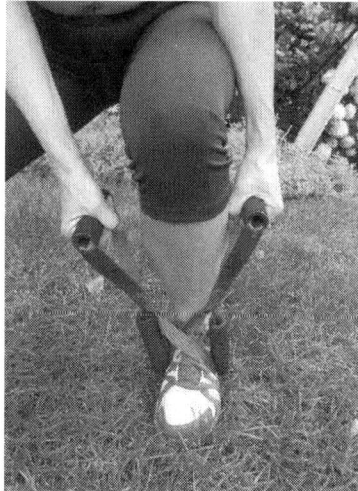

Legs – Upper Thighs

Iso-Bow® Side Leg Lunge - Left and Right Leg

Place the looped ends of two Iso-Bows® around the foot as shown to make a double stirrup. Bend the knee of that leg to about 90 degrees, while at the same

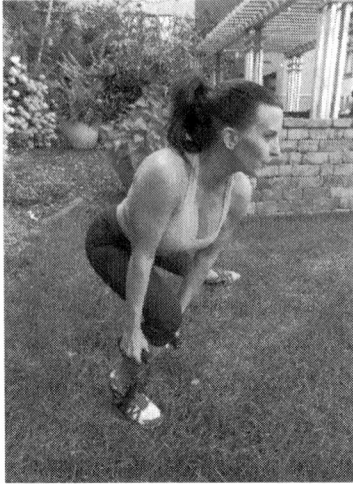

time moving the other leg out sideways, to create a side leg-lunge position.

Hold both Iso-Bow® handles firmly, and keeping your body upright and your back straight, use and engage the thigh and glute muscles of your leading leg as you attempt to straighten it and push upwards.

Breathe naturally and deeply in and out for about 10 full breaths, which will take about 1 second per breath.

Aim to perform an exercise breathing count of no less than

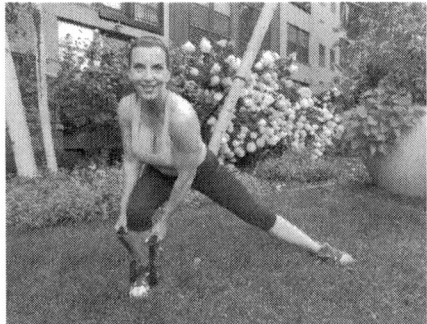

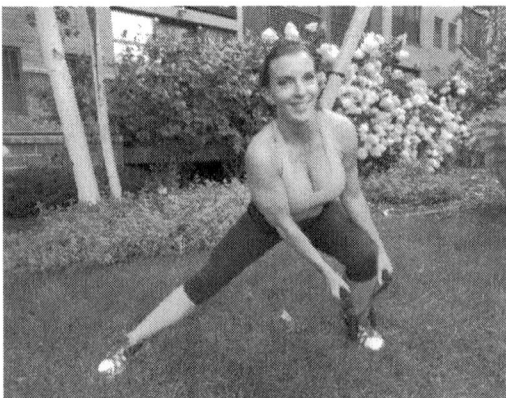

7 seconds, and for no longer than 10 seconds. Repeat the exercise with the other leg.

Iso-Bow® Forward Lunge - Left and Right Leg

Place the looped ends of two Iso-Bows® around the foot as shown to make a double stirrup.

Bend the knee to about 90 degrees, while at the same time move the other leg backwards, with your trailing knee close to the floor, to create a leg-lunge position.

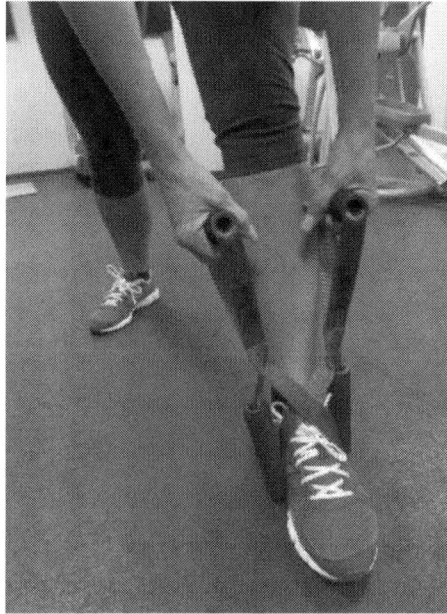

Hold both Iso-Bow® handles firmly, and keeping your body upright and your back straight, use and engage the thigh

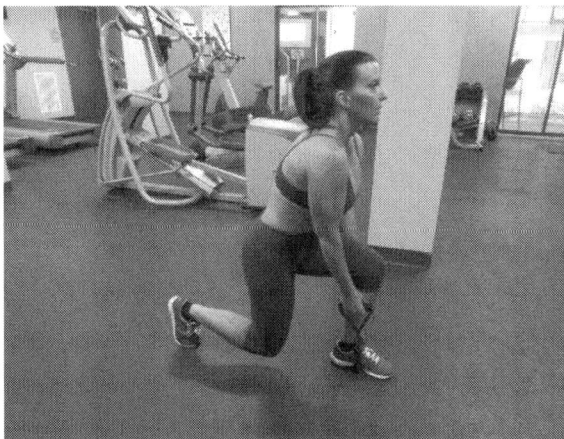

and glute muscles of your leading leg as you attempt to straighten it and push upwards.

Breathe naturally and deeply in and out for about 10 full breaths, which will take about 1 second per breath.

Aim to perform an exercise breathing count of no less than 7 seconds, and for no longer than 10 seconds. Repeat the exercise with the other leg.

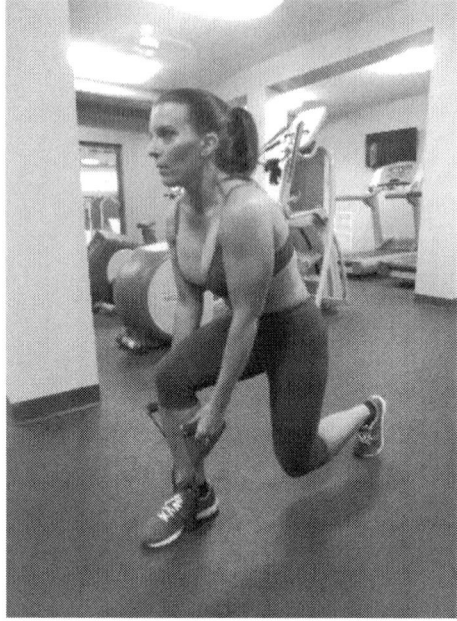

Standing Hamstring Wall Curl – Left and Right Leg

Stand with your back against a solid wall, or door which you can press your foot against. If you're using a vehicle you can use the wheel and tyre ('tire' in American vernacular) as a foot engagement point.

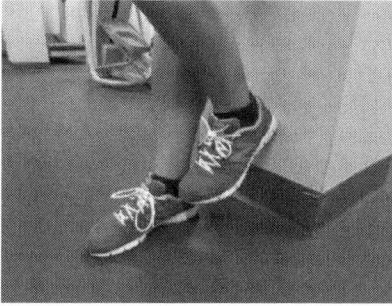

Bend one knee and place the heel of that leg against the wall, door, or vehicle to engage the hamstring muscles. Attempt to raise the heel as you press against the immovable object, and stabilize yourself with the other leg positioned slightly forwards to help you push backwards, and with an Iso-Bow® in front of you.

Breathe naturally and deeply in and out for about 10 full breaths, which will take about 1 second per breath. Aim to perform an exercise breathing count of no less than 7 seconds, and for no longer than 10 seconds. Repeat the exercise for the other leg, by swapping the leg and foot positions.

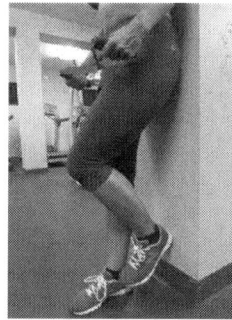

Breathe naturally and deeply in and out for about 10 full breaths, which will take about 1 second per breath.

Aim to perform an exercise breathing count of no less than 7 seconds, and for no longer than 10 seconds. Repeat the exercise for the other leg, by swapping the leg and foot positions.

Calf's

Calf Single Leg Wall Push – Left and Right Leg

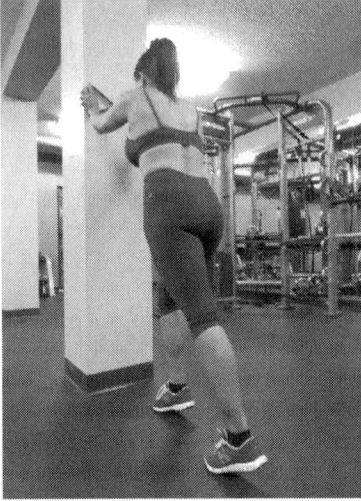

Hold an Iso-Bow® for balance, and place it together with your hands against a wall, a car, a door frame, or any other solid object which is immovable by human muscle power alone.

With one leg behind you in a firm position, and with the ball of your foot on the floor, raise the heel slightly as you engage your calf muscles, pushing against the immovable object.

Breathe naturally and deeply in and out for about 10 full breaths, which will take about 1 second per breath.

Aim to perform an exercise breathing count of no less than 7 seconds, and for no longer than 10 seconds.

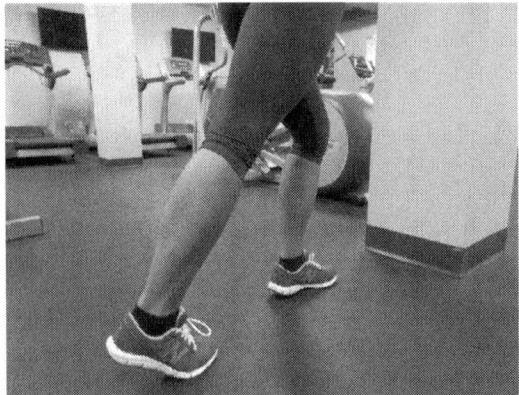

Switch legs and repeat the exercise with the other leg.

197

Upper Back

Dual Iso-Bow® Seated Foot-Stirrup Row

Sit upright on the floor, or on a chair, car seat or bench with your legs in front of you, bending your knees and hips, keeping the back straight at all times.

Place one looped end of each Iso-Bow® around each foot, hold the handles firmly and pull your elbows and arms back to engage your upper back muscles, being sure to keep your elbows close to your body as you do so.

Breathe naturally and deeply in and out for about 10 full breaths, which will take about 1 second per breath.

Aim to perform an exercise breathing count of no less than 7 seconds, and for no longer than 10 seconds.

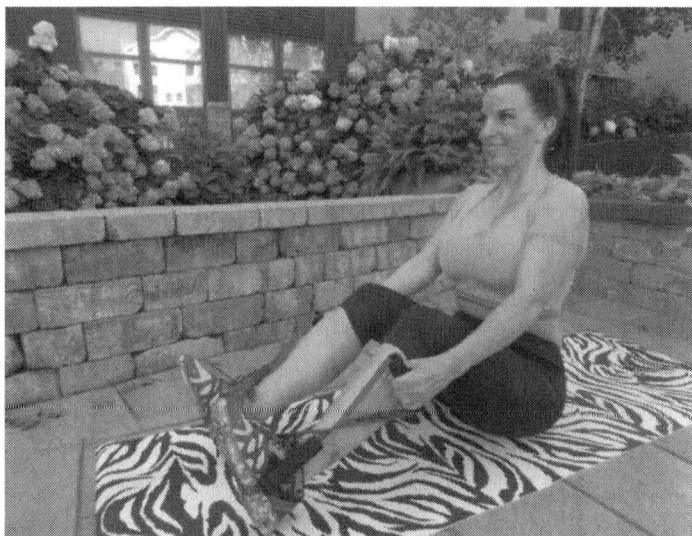

Chest

Dual Iso-Bow® Power Push

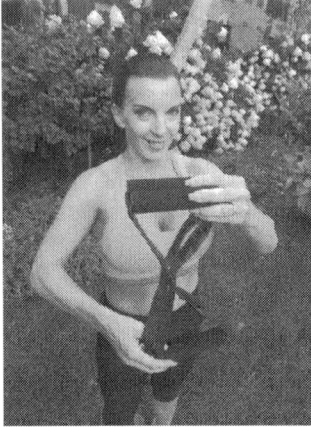

Wrap two Iso-Bows® together as shown, and hold the 4 combined handles, in a comfortable and firm position with the handles sitting low in the palms of each hand, near to the wrists.

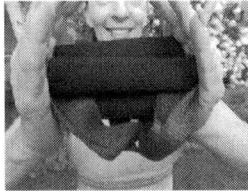

Press the combined Iso-Bows® together to engage your chest muscles, with your arms

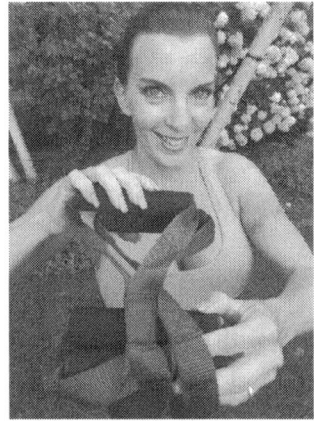

roughly parallel to the floor as you attempt to compress the immovable handles. Breathe naturally and deeply in and out for about 10 full breaths, which will take about 1 second per breath.

Aim to perform an exercise breathing count of no less than 7 seconds, and for no longer than 10 seconds.

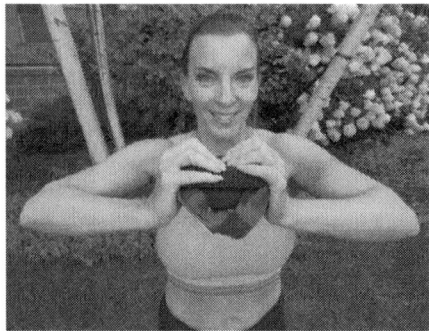

199

Shoulders

Iso-Bow® Single Arm Overhead Press – Left and Right Arm

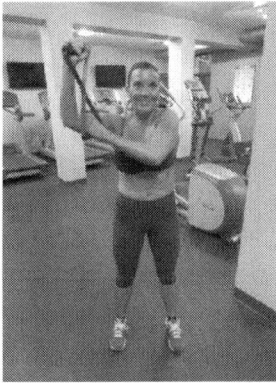

Place one arm so that it's out and to the side, approximately parallel to the floor. Hold one end of the Iso-Bow®, and ensure that your upper arm stays at an angle of approximately 90-degrees at all times.

Push upwards as if to perform a shoulder press, and resist the movement by pulling back and downwards with the opposing hand and arm.

Breathe naturally and deeply in and out for about 10 full

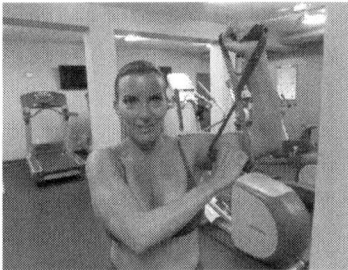

breaths, which will take about 1 second per breath.

Aim to perform an exercise breathing count of no less than 7 seconds, and for no

longer than 10 seconds.

Then repeat the exercise on the other side by reversing the hand and arm positions.

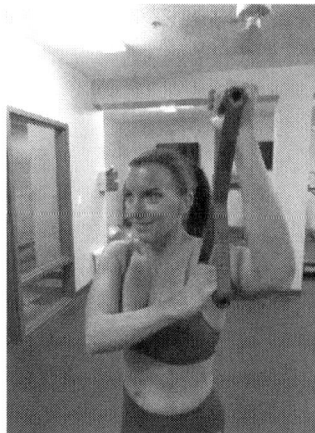

Iso-Bow® Mid Hold Lateral Pull Apart - AKA Lateral Raise

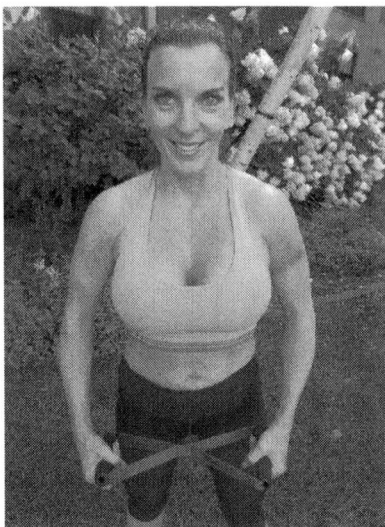

Hold the Iso-Bow® in both hands, at lap level in front of you, and with your elbows very slightly bent. In this position, attempt to pull it apart by raising both arms sideways, and engaging the side shoulder muscles as you do so.

Breathe naturally and deeply in and out for about 10 full breaths, which will take about 1 second per breath.

Aim to perform an exercise breathing count of no less than 7 seconds, and for no longer than 10 seconds.

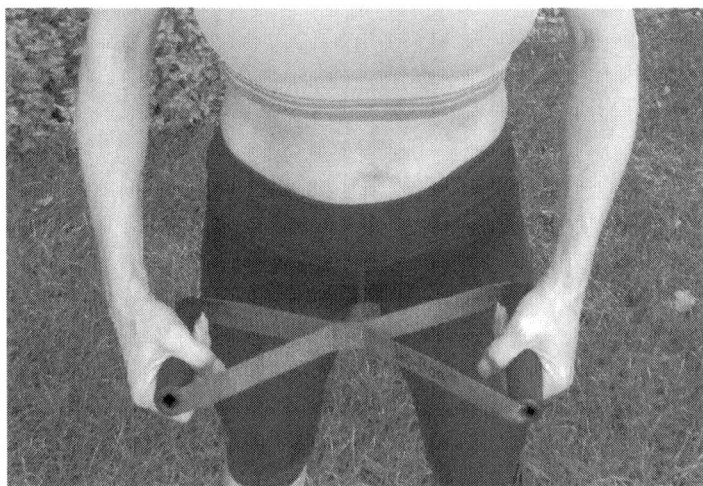

Arms – Biceps and Triceps

Iso-Bow® Single Arms Biceps Curl – Left and Right Arm

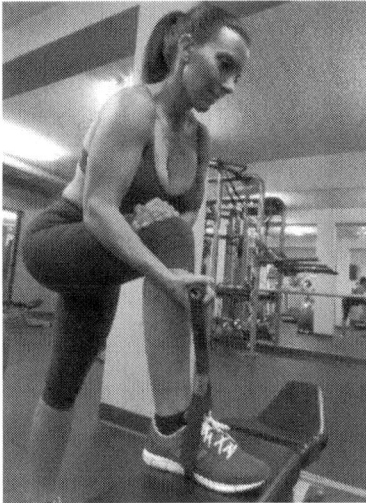

Form a loop on one side of the Iso-Bow® handle as shown, place it around your left foot, and put your left foot on a solid object such as bench or a chair.

Lean forward and grip the Iso-Bow® handle with your left hand facing

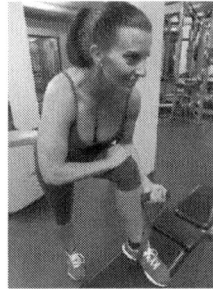

up, bracing yourself with your free hand against the bent knee.

Try to pull the Iso-Bow® up to engage the biceps muscles, with your foot

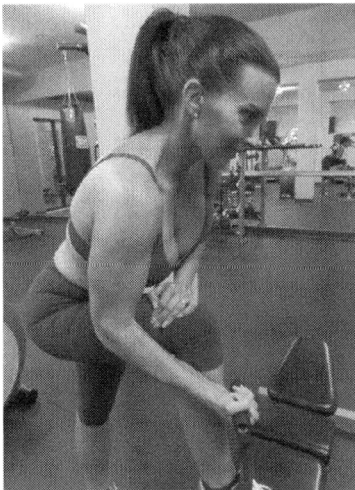

resisting the exercise.

Breathe naturally and deeply in and out for about 10 full breaths, which will take about 1 second per breath. Aim to perform an exercise breathing count of no less than 7 seconds, and for no longer than 10 seconds.

Iso-Bow® Triceps Press Down Over Knee

Put one foot on a solid object such as bench or a chair, and place the Iso-Bow® in a comfortable position face downwards, close to the knee and hold both handles.

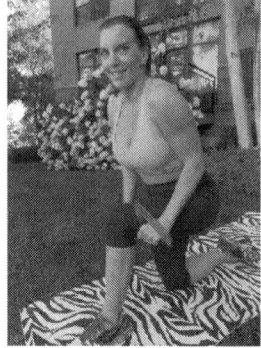

Bend the arms and learn forwards over the knee, and keeping your elbows close to your body at all times while pushing down on each handle to engage the triceps muscles of both arms as you attempt to push your body back into an upright position.

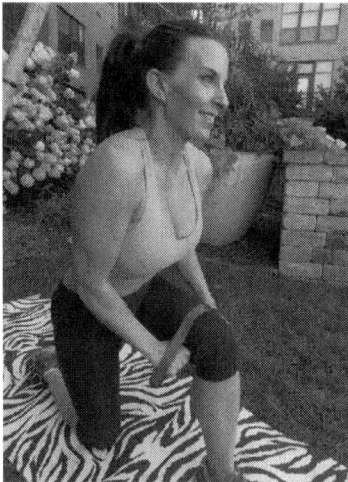

You won't be able to move, because your bodyweight and your upper body muscles will prevent you.

Breathe naturally and deeply in and out for about 10 full breaths, which will take about 1 second per breath.

Aim to perform an exercise breathing count of no less than 7 seconds, and for no longer than 10 seconds.

Aim to perform an exercise breathing count of no less than 7 seconds, and for no longer than 10 seconds.

Forearms

Iso-Bow® Seated Wrist Curl and Extension

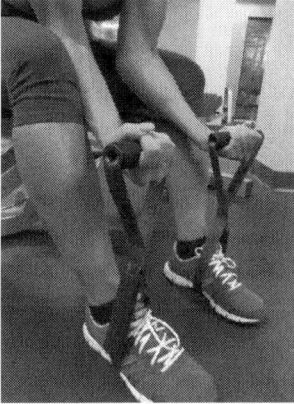

Place an Iso-Bow® around each foot, and hold both handles with your palms facing up, attempt to curl both wrists upwards, to engage the forearm muscles.

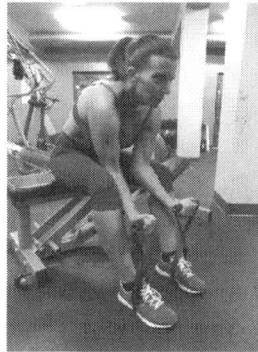

Breathe naturally and deeply in and out for about 10 full breaths, which

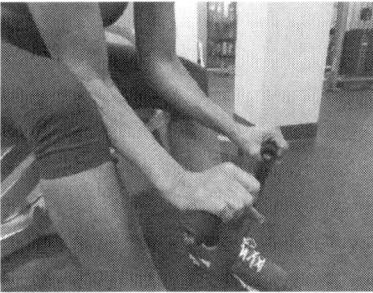

will take about 1 second per breath.

Aim to perform an exercise breathing count of no less than 7 seconds, and for no longer than 10 seconds. Switch your grip so that your palms are facing down, and repeat the exercise.

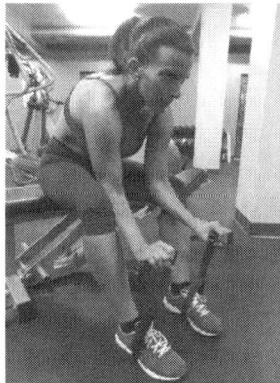

Lower Back

Dual Iso-Bow® Bent Leg Deadlift

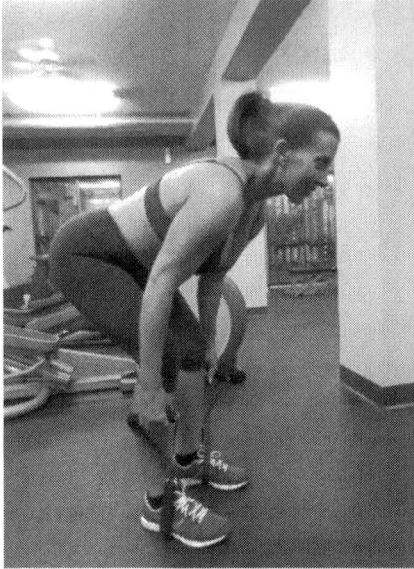

Place the loop handle of both Iso-Bows® around each foot as shown. Hold each handle firmly while maintaining a perfect bent-knee, semi squat position with your back straight at all times, then attempt to slowly stand up straight.

Engage the muscles of the glutes, hamstrings, lower back, thighs, and other core muscles, while the Iso-

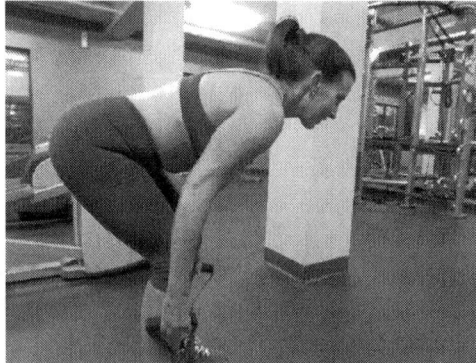

Bows® secured by your feet prevent any movement from taking place.

Breathe naturally and deeply in and out for about 10 full breaths, which will take about 1 second per breath.

Aim to perform an exercise breathing count of no less than 7 seconds, and for no longer than 10 seconds.

Abdominals

Iso-Bow® V-Sit Side to Side

Lay down, and raise your legs and torso off the floor by curling the spine, gripping the Iso-Bow® securely with both hands close to your mid-section.

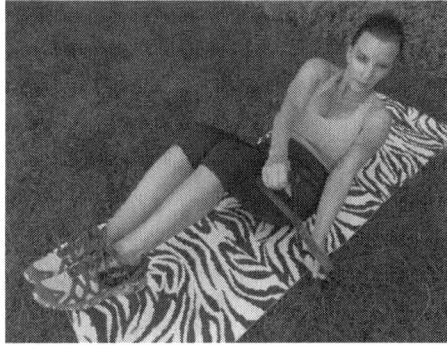

Twist the Iso-Bow® to one side as you engage the abdominal and oblique muscles.

Breathe naturally and deeply in and out for about 10 full breaths, which will take about 1 second per breath.

Aim to perform an exercise breathing count of no less than 7 seconds, and for no longer than 10 seconds. Repeat the exercise on the other side of your body.

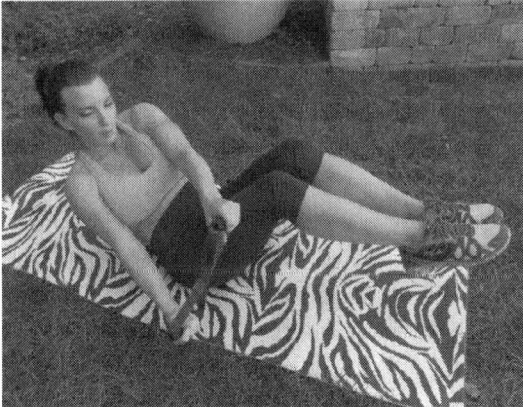

The ISO90™ Course Week 10 at a Glance

Legs – Upper Thighs

- △ *Iso-Bow® Side Leg Lunge - Left and Right Leg*
- △ *Iso-Bow® Forward Lunge - Left and Right Leg*
- △ *Standing Hamstring Wall Curl – Left and Right Leg*

Calf's

- △ *Calf Single Leg Wall Push – Left and Right Leg*

Upper Back

- △ *Dual Iso-Bow® Seated Foot-Stirrup Row*

Chest

- △ *Dual Iso-Bow® Power Push*

Shoulders

- △ *Iso-Bow® Single Arm Overhead Press – Left and Right Arm*
- △ *Iso-Bow® Mid Hold Lateral Pull Apart - AKA Lateral Raise*

Arms – Biceps and Triceps

- △ *Iso-Bow® Single Arms Biceps Curl – Left and Right Arm*
- △ *Iso-Bow® Triceps Press Down Over Knee*

Forearms

- △ *Iso-Bow® Seated Wrist Curl and Extension*

Lower Back

- △ *Dual Iso-Bow® Bent Leg Deadlift*

Abdominals

- △ *Iso-Bow® V-Sit Side to Side*

The ISO90™ Course Week 11

Week 11 Notes

△ The same routine as week 10, while still to slightly increase the intensity used with all exercises, and reduce the amount of rest time in between.

△ Apply approximately 75% of your maximum potential intensity to each exercise.

Perform only one 7 second isometric exercise contraction. *(Don't start counting until you've fully applied the desired level of intensity)*

△ Before you begin the full isometric contraction part of the exercise, take between 2 and 3 additional seconds to perform Dynamic Flexation™ to help you properly engage the muscles and joints. Similarly, at the end of each isometric exercise, do the same in reverse as you disengage from the exercise over a period of between 2 and 3 seconds.

△ Perform the workout EVERY DAY with NO rest days.

△ Focus on perfect exercise form

Legs – Upper Thighs

Iso-Bow® Side Leg Lunge - Left and Right Leg

Place the looped ends of two Iso-Bows® around the foot as shown to make a double stirrup. Bend the knee of that leg to about 90 degrees, while at the same

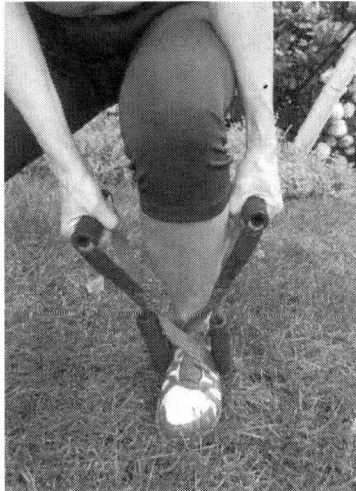

time moving the other leg out sideways, to create a side leg-lunge position.

Hold both Iso-Bow® handles firmly, and keeping your body upright and your back straight, use and engage the thigh and glute muscles of your leading leg as you attempt to straighten it and push upwards.

Breathe naturally and deeply in and out for about 10 full breaths, which will take about 1 second per breath.

Aim to perform an exercise breathing count of no less than

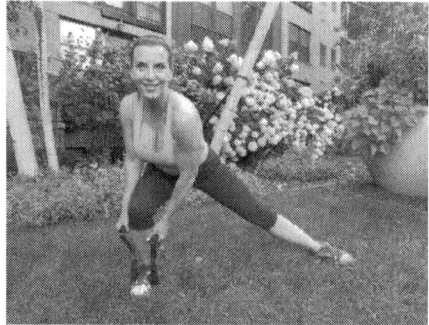

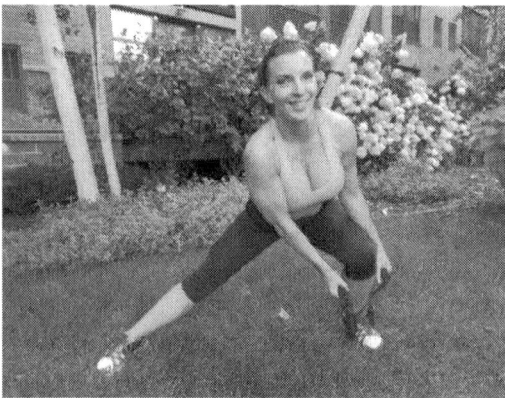

7 seconds, and for no longer than 10 seconds. Repeat the exercise with the other leg.

Iso-Bow® Forward Lunge - Left and Right Leg

Place the looped ends of two Iso-Bows® around the foot as shown to make a double stirrup.

Bend the knee to about 90 degrees, while at the same time move the other leg backwards, with your trailing knee close to the floor, to create a leg-lunge position.

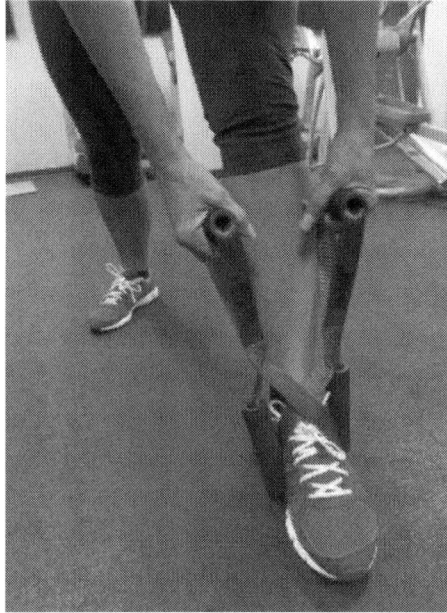

Hold both Iso-Bow® handles firmly, and keeping your body upright and your back straight, use and engage the thigh and glute muscles of your leading leg as you attempt to straighten it and push upwards.

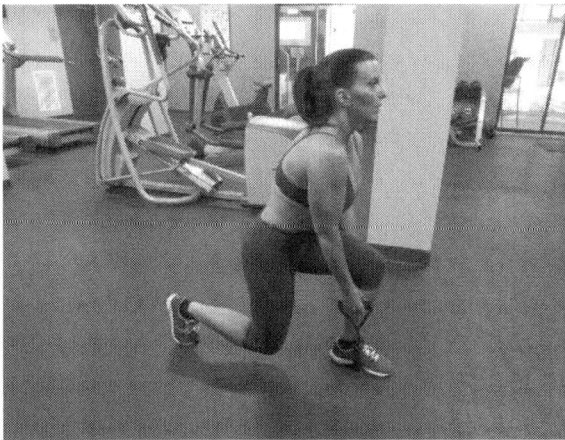

Breathe naturally and deeply in and out for about 10 full breaths, which will take about 1 second per breath.

Aim to perform an exercise breathing count of no less than 7 seconds, and for no longer than 10 seconds. Repeat the exercise with the other leg.

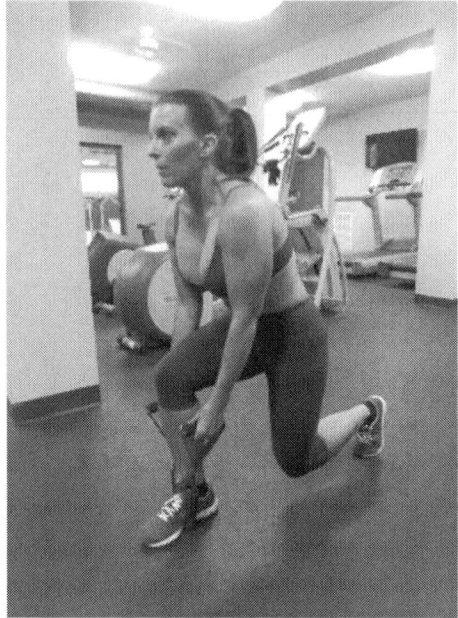

Standing Hamstring Wall Curl – Left and Right Leg

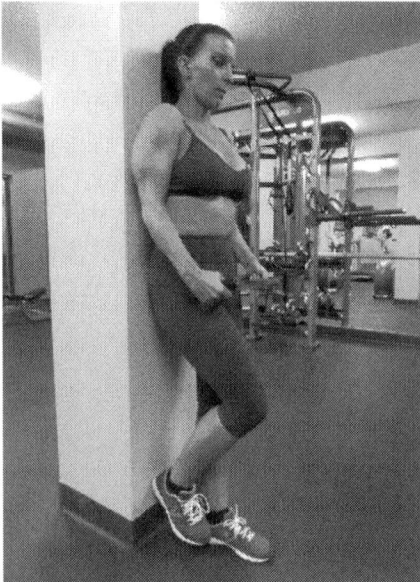

Stand with your back against a solid wall, or door which you can press your foot against. If you're using a vehicle you can use the wheel and tyre ('tire' in American vernacular) as a foot engagement point.

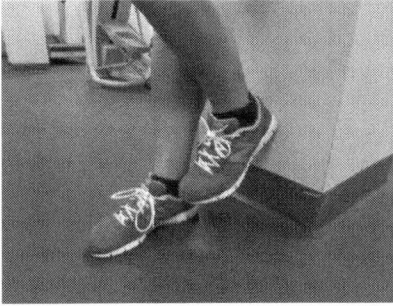

Bend one knee and place the heel of that leg against the wall, door, or vehicle to engage the hamstring muscles. Attempt to raise the heel as you press against the immovable object, and stabilize yourself with the other leg positioned slightly forwards to help you push backwards, and with an Iso-Bow® in front of you.

Breathe naturally and deeply in and out for about 10 full breaths, which will take about 1 second per breath. Aim to perform an exercise breathing count of no less than 7 seconds, and for no longer than 10 seconds. Repeat the exercise for the other leg, by swapping the leg and foot positions.

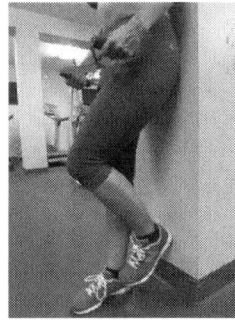

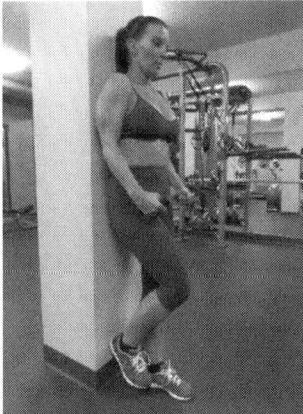

Breathe naturally and deeply in and out for about 10 full breaths, which will take about 1 second per breath.

Aim to perform an exercise breathing count of no less than 7 seconds, and for no longer than 10 seconds. Repeat the exercise for the other leg, by swapping the leg and foot positions.

Calf's

Calf Single Leg Wall Push - Left and Right Leg

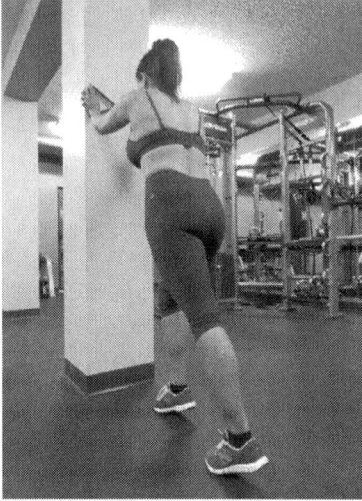

Hold an Iso-Bow® for balance, and place it together with your hands against a wall, a car, a door frame, or any other solid object which is immovable by human muscle power alone.

With one leg behind you in a firm position, and with the ball of your foot on the floor, raise the heel slightly as you engage your calf muscles, pushing against the immovable object.

Breathe naturally and deeply in and out for about 10 full breaths, which will take about 1 second per breath.

Aim to perform an exercise breathing count of no less than 7 seconds, and for no longer than 10 seconds.

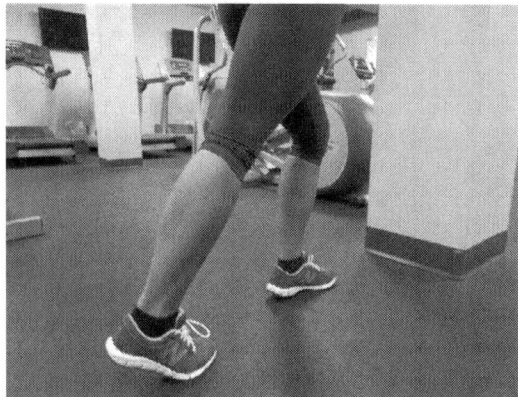

Switch legs and repeat the exercise with the other leg.

Upper Back

Dual Iso-Bow® Seated Foot-Stirrup Row

Sit upright on the floor, or on a chair, car seat or bench with your legs in front of you, bending your knees and hips, keeping the back straight at all times.

Place one looped end of each Iso-Bow® around each foot, hold the handles firmly and pull your elbows and arms back to engage your upper back muscles, being sure to keep your elbows close to your body as you do so.

Breathe naturally and deeply in and out for about 10 full breaths, which will take about 1 second per breath.

Aim to perform an exercise breathing count of no less than 7 seconds, and for no longer than 10 seconds.

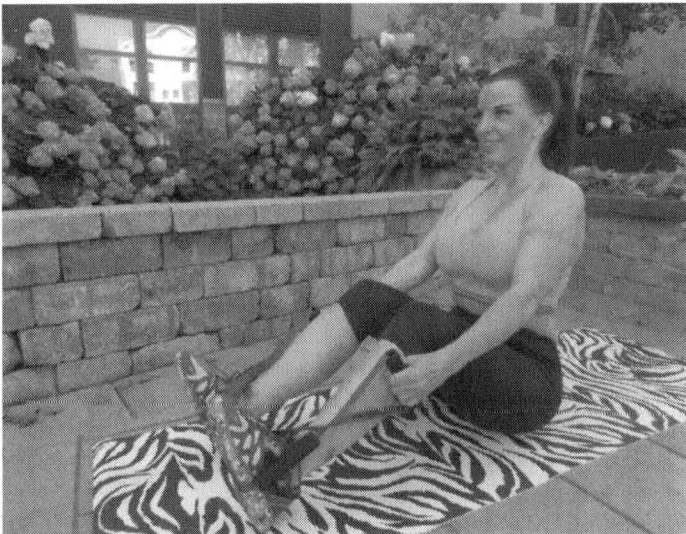

Chest

Dual Iso-Bow® Power Push

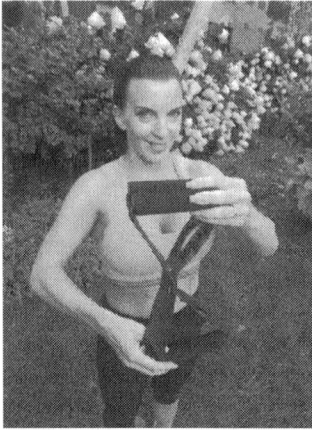

Wrap two Iso-Bows® together as shown, and hold the 4 combined handles, in a comfortable and firm position with the handles sitting low in the palms of each hand, near to the wrists.

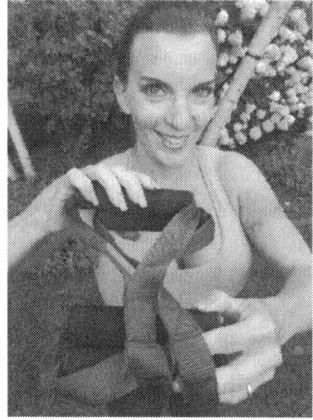

Press the combined Iso-Bows® together engage your chest muscles, with your arms

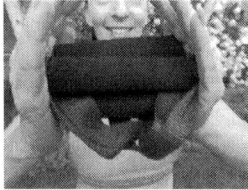

roughly parallel to the floor as you attempt to compress the immovable handles. Breathe naturally and deeply in and out for about 10 full breaths, which will take about 1 second per breath.

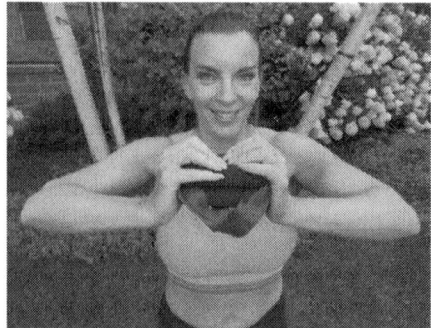

Aim to perform an exercise breathing count of no less than 7 seconds, and for no longer than 10 seconds.

Shoulders

Iso-Bow® Single Arm Overhead Press – Left and Right Arm

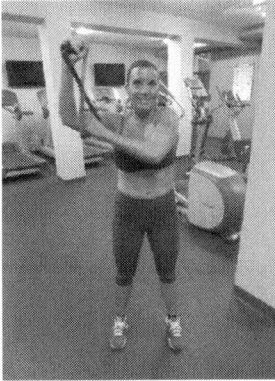

Place one arm so that it's out and to the side, approximately parallel to the floor. Hold one end of the Iso-Bow®, and ensure that your upper arm stays at an angle of approximately 90-degrees at all times.

Push upwards as if to perform a shoulder press, and resist the movement by pulling back and downwards with the opposing hand and arm.

Breathe naturally and deeply in and out for about 10 full breaths, which will take about 1 second per breath.

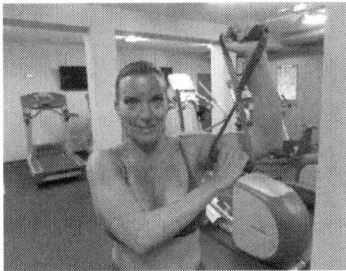

Aim to perform an exercise breathing count of no less than 7 seconds, and for no longer than 10 seconds.

Then repeat the exercise on the other side by reversing the hand and arm positions.

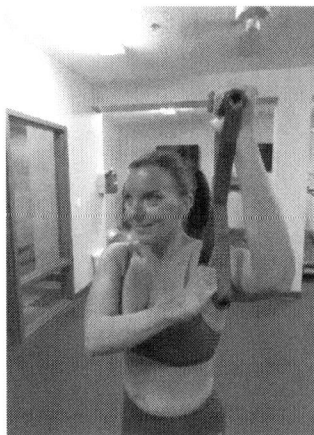

Iso-Bow® Mid Hold Lateral Pull Apart - AKA Lateral Raise

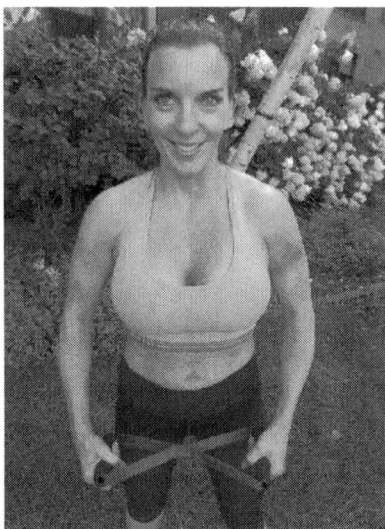

Hold the Iso-Bow® in both hands, at lap level in front of you, and with your elbows very slightly bent. In this position, attempt to pull it apart by raising both arms sideways, and engaging the side shoulder muscles as you do so.

Breathe naturally and deeply in and out for about 10 full breaths, which will take about 1 second per breath.

Aim to perform an exercise breathing count of no less than 7 seconds, and for no longer than 10 seconds.

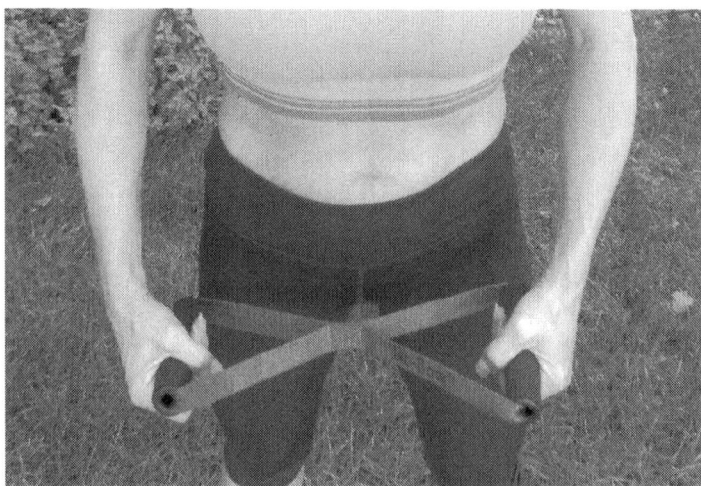

Arms – Biceps and Triceps

Iso-Bow® Single Arms Biceps Curl – Left and Right Arm

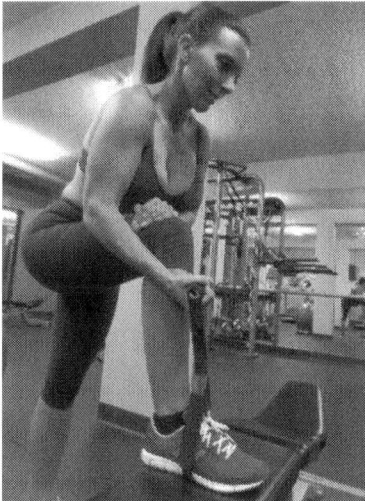

Form a loop on one side of the Iso-Bow® handle as shown, place it around your left foot, and put your left foot on a solid object such as bench or a chair.

Lean forward and grip the Iso-Bow® handle with your left hand facing up, bracing yourself with your free hand against the bent knee.

Try to pull the Iso-Bow® up to engage the biceps muscles, with your foot resisting the exercise.

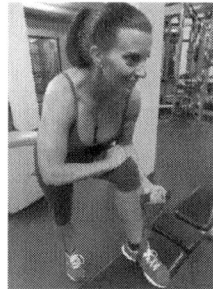

Breathe naturally and deeply in and out for about 10 full breaths, which will take about 1 second per breath. Aim to perform an exercise breathing count of no less than 7 seconds, and for no longer than 10 seconds.

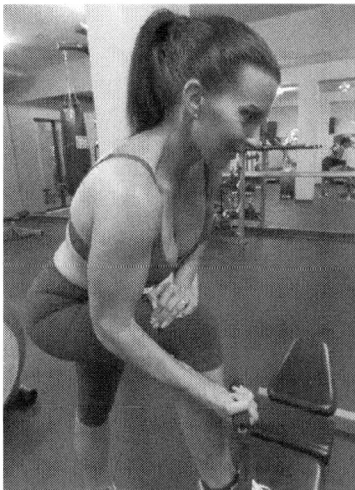

Iso-Bow® Triceps Press Down Over Knee

Put one foot on a solid object such as bench or a chair, and place the Iso-Bow® in a comfortable position face downwards, close to the knee and hold both handles.

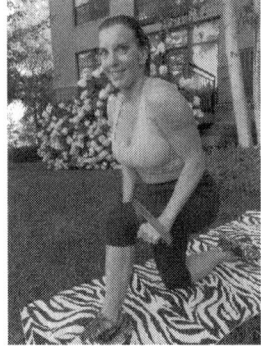

Bend the arms and learn forwards over the knee, and keeping your elbows close to your body at all times while pushing down on each handle to engage the triceps muscles of both arms as you attempt to push your body back into an upright position.

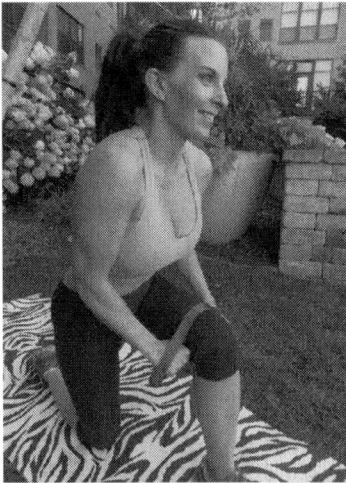

You won't be able to move, because your bodyweight and your upper body muscles will prevent you.

Breathe naturally and deeply in and out for about 10 full breaths, which will take about 1 second per breath.

Aim to perform an exercise breathing count of no less than 7 seconds, and for no longer than 10 seconds.

Aim to perform an exercise breathing count of no less than 7 seconds, and for no longer than 10 seconds.

Forearms

Iso-Bow® Seated Wrist Curl and Extension

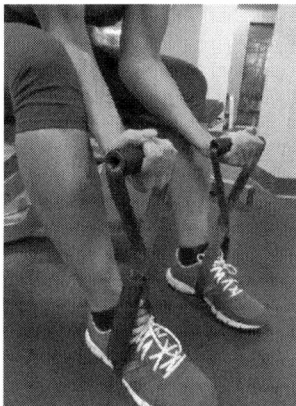

Place an Iso-Bow® around each foot, and hold both handles with your palms facing up, attempt to curl both wrists upwards, to engage the forearm muscles.

Breathe naturally and deeply in and out for about 10 full breaths, which

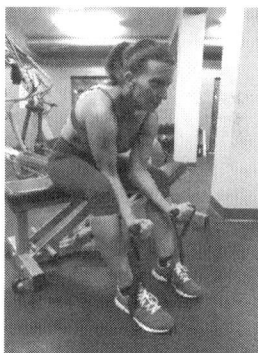

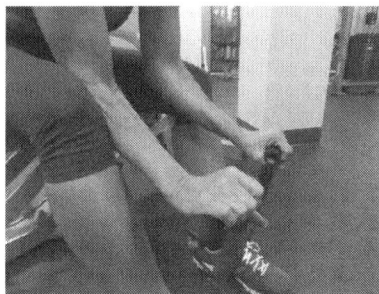

will take about 1 second per breath.

Aim to perform an exercise breathing count of no less than 7 seconds, and for no longer than 10 seconds. Switch your grip so that your palms are facing down, and repeat the exercise.

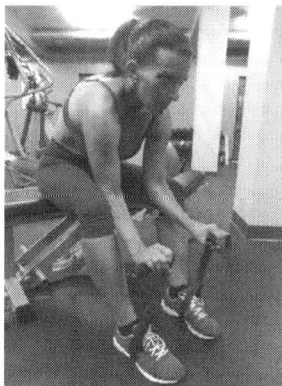

Lower Back

Dual Iso-Bow® Bent Leg Deadlift

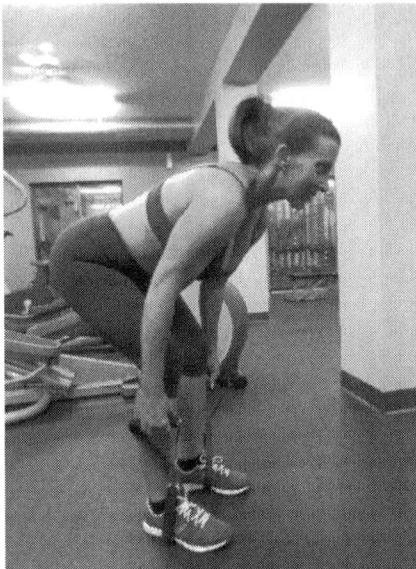

Place the loop handle of both Iso-Bows® around each foot as shown. Hold each handle firmly while maintaining a perfect bent-knee, semi squat position with your back straight at all times, then attempt to slowly stand up straight.

Engage the muscles of the glutes, hamstrings, lower back, thighs, and other core muscles, while the Iso-

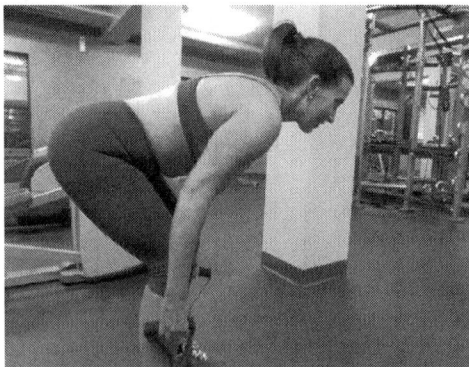

Bows® secured by your feet prevent any movement from taking place.

Breathe naturally and deeply in and out for about 10 full breaths, which will take about 1 second per breath.

Aim to perform an exercise breathing count of no less than 7 seconds, and for no longer than 10 seconds.

Abdominals

Iso-Bow® V-Sit Side to Side

Lay down, and raise your legs and torso off the floor by curling the spine, gripping the Iso-Bow® securely with both hands close to your mid-section.

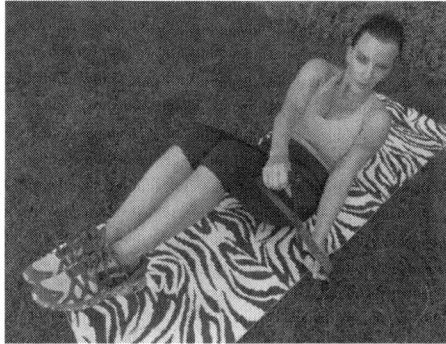

Twist the Iso-Bow® to one side as you engage the abdominal and oblique muscles.

Breathe naturally and deeply in and out for about 10 full breaths, which will take about 1 second per breath.

Aim to perform an exercise breathing count of no less than 7 seconds, and for no longer than 10 seconds. Repeat the exercise on the other side of your body.

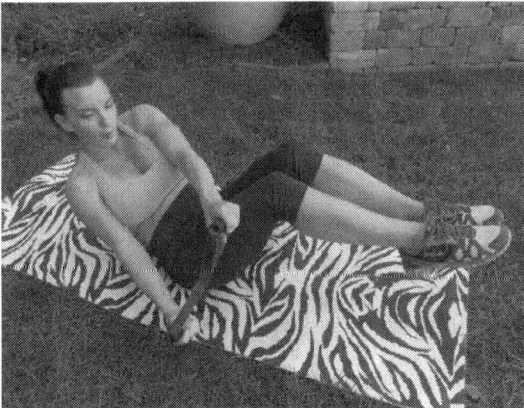

The ISO90™ Course Week 11 at a Glance

Legs – Upper Thighs

- △ Iso-Bow® Side Leg Lunge - Left and Right Leg
- △ Iso-Bow® Forward Lunge - Left and Right Leg
- △ Standing Hamstring Wall Curl – Left and Right Leg

Calf's

- △ Calf Single Leg Wall Push - Left and Right Leg

Upper Back

- △ Dual Iso-Bow® Seated Foot-Stirrup Row

Chest

- △ Dual Iso-Bow® Power Push

Shoulders

- △ Iso-Bow® Single Arm Overhead Press – Left and Right Arm
- △ Iso-Bow® Mid Hold Lateral Pull Apart - AKA Lateral Raise

Arms – Biceps and Triceps

- △ Iso-Bow® Single Arms Biceps Curl – Left and Right Arm
- △ Iso-Bow® Triceps Press Down Over Knee

Forearms

- △ Iso-Bow® Seated Wrist Curl and Extension

Lower Back

- △ Dual Iso-Bow® Bent Leg Deadlift

Abdominals

- △ Iso-Bow® V-Sit Side to Side

223

The ISO90™ Course Week 12

Week 12 Notes

- △ NEW routine. Apply even more intensity to all exercises, and try to further reduce the amount of rest time between exercises.
- △ Apply approximately 75-80% of your maximum potential intensity to each exercise.

Perform only one 7 second isometric exercise contraction. *(Don't start counting until you've fully applied the desired level of intensity)*

- △ Before you begin the full isometric contraction part of the exercise, take between 2 and 3 additional seconds to perform Dynamic Flexation™ to help you properly engage the muscles and joints. Similarly, at the end of each isometric exercise, do the same in reverse as you disengage from the exercise over a period of between 2 and 3 seconds.
- △ Perform the workout EVERY DAY with NO rest days.

Legs – Upper Thighs

Dual Iso-Bow® Stirrup Squat

Place the looped handle side of each Iso-Bow® around each foot as shown. Bend your knees deeply to assume the squat position, bending your torso only at

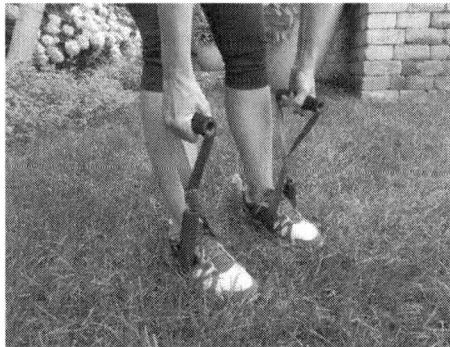

the hips, and keeping your back straight and upright at all times.

Grip each Iso-Bow® handle firmly, and attempt to stand up straight by engaging your upper thigh and glute muscles. Naturally you won't be able to move, but continue your attempt to stand up, while maintain the perfect mid-squat position as you do so.

Breathe naturally and deeply in and out for about 10 full breaths, which will take about 1 second per breath.

Aim to perform an exercise breathing count of no less than 7 seconds, and for no longer than 10 seconds.

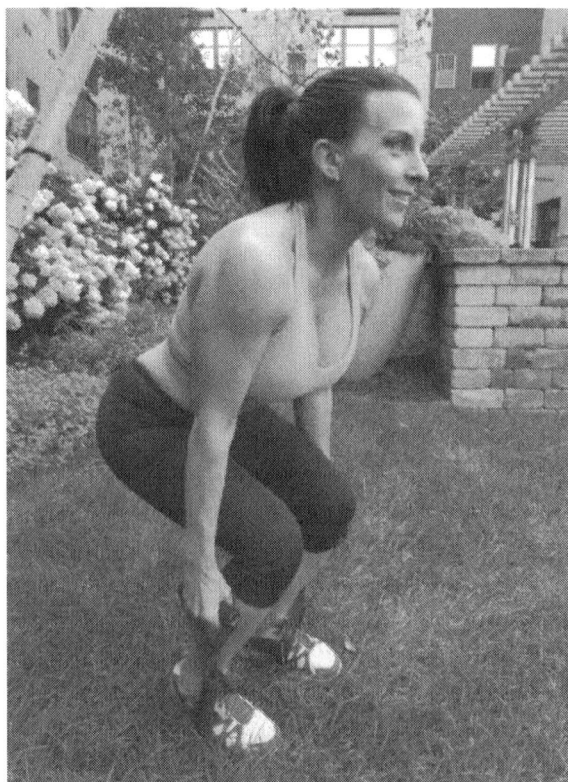

Standing Hamstring Wall Curl – Left and Right Leg

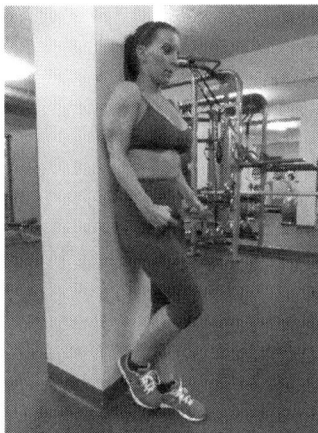

Stand with your back against a solid wall, or door which you can press your foot against. If you're using a vehicle you can use the wheel and tyre ('tire' in American vernacular) as a foot engagement point.

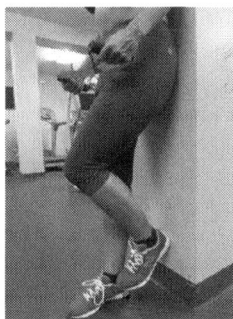

Bend one knee and place the heel of that leg against the wall, door, or vehicle to engage the hamstring muscles. Attempt to raise the heel as you press against the immovable object, and stabilize yourself with the other

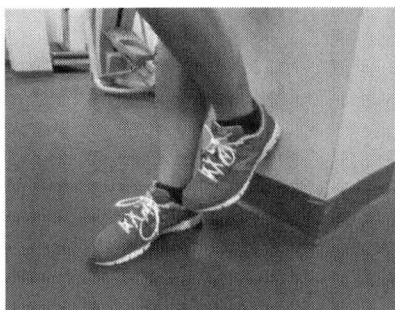

leg positioned slightly forwards to help you push backwards, and with an Iso-Bow® in front of you.

Breathe naturally and deeply in and out for about 10 full breaths, which will take about 1 second per breath. Aim to perform an exercise breathing count of no less than 7 seconds, and for no longer than 10 seconds. Repeat the exercise for the other leg, by swapping the leg and foot positions.

226

Calf's

Calf Single Leg Wall Push – Left and Right Leg

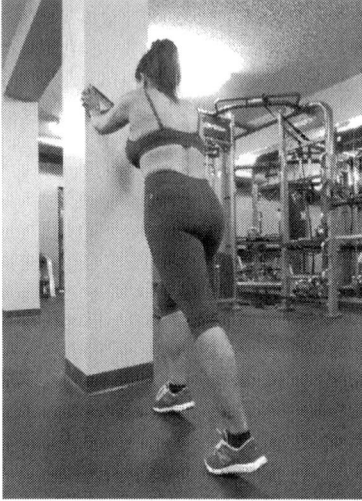

Hold an Iso-Bow® for balance, and place it together with your hands against a wall, a car, a door frame, or any other solid object which is immovable by human muscle power alone.

With one leg behind you in a firm position, and with the ball of your foot on the floor, raise the heel slightly as you engage your calf muscles, pushing against the immovable object.

Breathe naturally and deeply in and out for about 10 full breaths, which will take about 1 second per breath.

Aim to perform an exercise breathing count of no less than 7 seconds, and for no longer than 10 seconds.

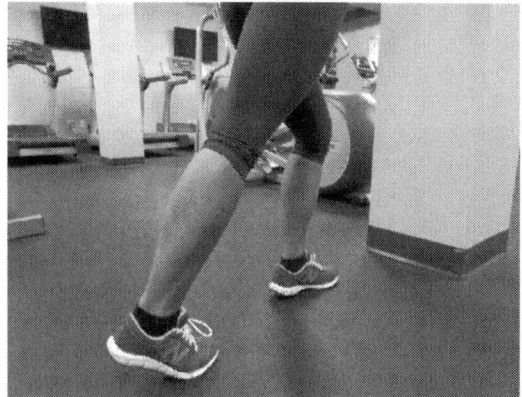

Switch legs and repeat the exercise with the other leg.

Upper Back

Iso-Bow® Doorway Pull Ups

Place one handle of each Iso-Bow® over the top of a solid door as shown, at about shoulder width apart, close the door, and double check that it's secure.

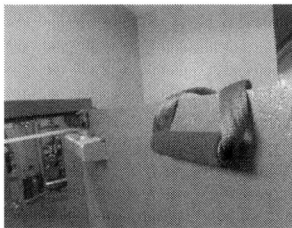

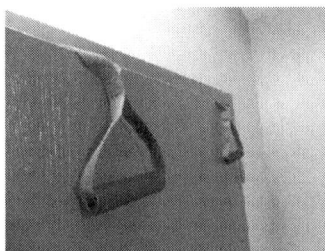

Holding each handle, pull yourself up so that you slide up against the door, until your elbows are bent at about a 90-degree angle. Hold this position to engage the upper back muscles as you attempt to pull upwards and forwards as you press against the door which will prevent you from moving.

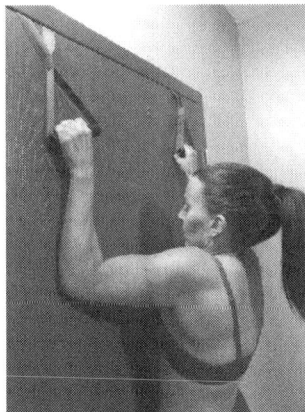

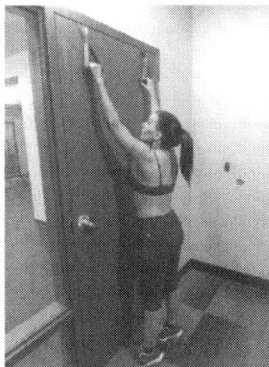

Breathe naturally and deeply in and out for about 10 full breaths, which will take about 1 second per breath. Aim to perform an exercise breathing count of no less than 7 seconds, and for no longer than 10 seconds.

ONLY PERFORM IF IT IS SAFE TO DO SO ON A SOLID DOOR.

Upper Back - Alternative to Pull Ups

Dual Iso-Bow® Seated Foot-Stirrup Row

Sit upright on the floor, or on a chair, car seat or bench with your legs in front of you, bending your knees and hips, keeping the back straight at all times.

Place one looped end of each Iso-Bow® around each foot, hold the handles firmly and pull your elbows and arms back to engage your upper back muscles, being sure to keep your elbows close to your body as you do so.

Breathe naturally and deeply in and out for about 10 full breaths, which will take about 1 second per breath.

Aim to perform an exercise breathing count of no less than 7 seconds, and for no longer than 10 seconds.

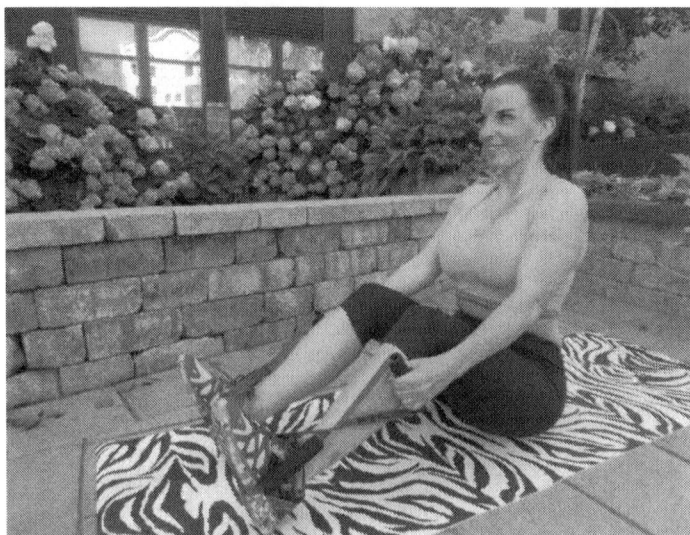

Chest

Iso-Bow® Chest Press and Upper Back Row – Left and Right

With one arm in front of you roughly parallel to the

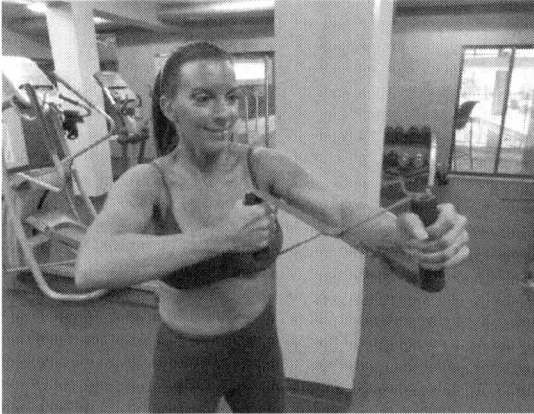

floor, push one end of the Iso-Bow® forwards, and at the same time pull the other handle backwards, keep the elbows of both arms slightly bent at all times.

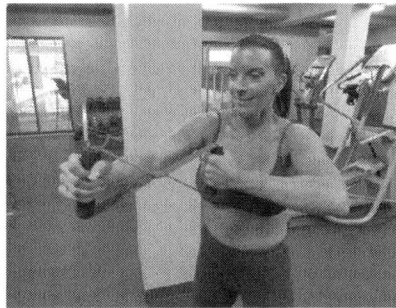

Breathe naturally and deeply in and out for about 10 full breaths, which will take about 1 second per breath.

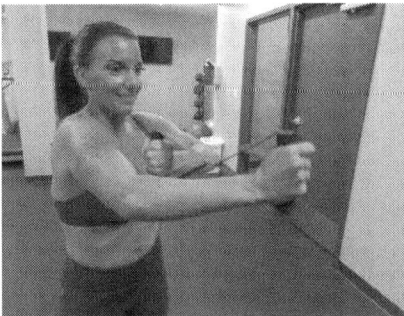

Aim to perform an exercise breathing count of no less than 7 seconds, and for no longer than 10 seconds.

Shoulders

Iso-Bow® Single Arm Overhead Press – Left and Right Arm

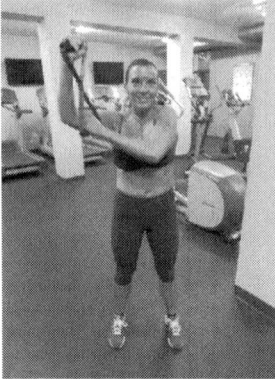

Place one arm so that it's out and to the side, approximately parallel to the floor. Hold one end of the Iso-Bow®, and ensure that your upper arm stays at an angle of approximately 90-degrees at all times.

Push upwards as if to perform a shoulder press, and resist the movement by pulling back and downwards with the opposing hand and arm.

Breathe naturally and deeply in and out for about 10 full

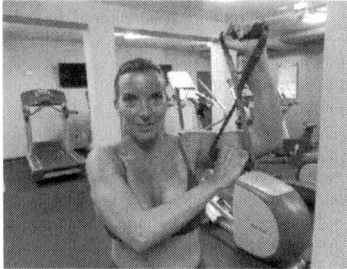

breaths, which will take about 1 second per breath.

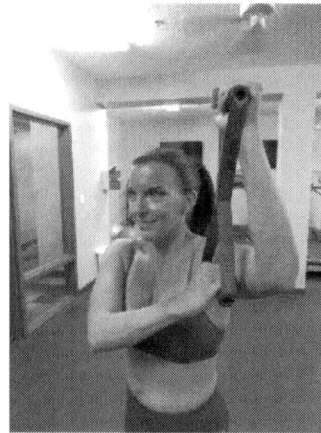

Aim to perform an exercise breathing count of no less than 7 seconds, and for no longer than 10 seconds.

Then repeat the exercise on the other side by reversing the hand and arm positions.

Iso-Bow® Mid Hold Lateral Pull Apart - AKA Lateral Raise

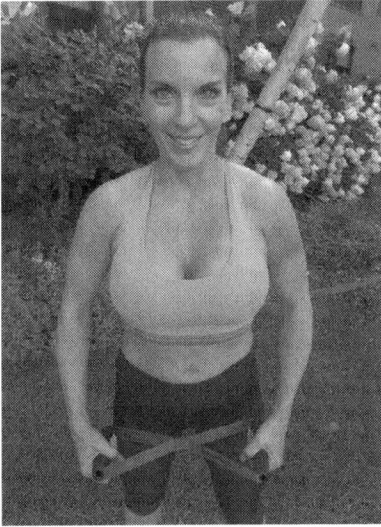

Hold the Iso-Bow® in both hands, at lap level in front of you, and with your elbows very slightly bent. In this position, attempt to pull it apart by raising both arms sideways, and engaging the side shoulder muscles as you do so.

Breathe naturally and deeply in and out for about 10 full breaths, which will take about 1 second per breath.

Aim to perform an exercise breathing count of no less than 7 seconds, and for no longer than 10 seconds.

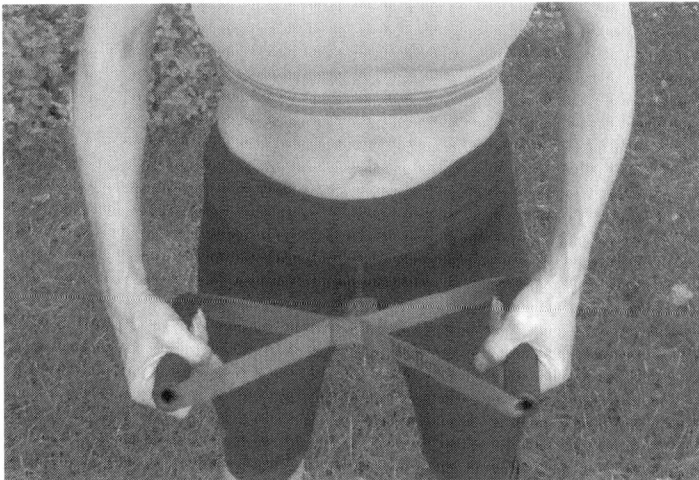

Arms

Iso-Bow® Biceps and Triceps Cradle Press-Curl (Left Side)

Firstly, you'll exercise the biceps of your right arm, and triceps muscles of your left arm.

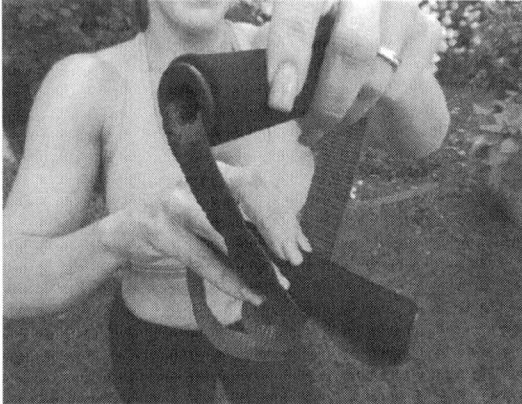

Cradle the Iso-Bow® with your left hand, gripping the top with your right hand facing up. Grip the cradled side of the Iso-Bow® with the left hand facing down.

Keep both elbows close to your body, and with your right arm across the front of you at waist height. In this position, press down with the left hand, and at the same time press up with the right, to engage both the Biceps and Triceps muscles simultaneously.

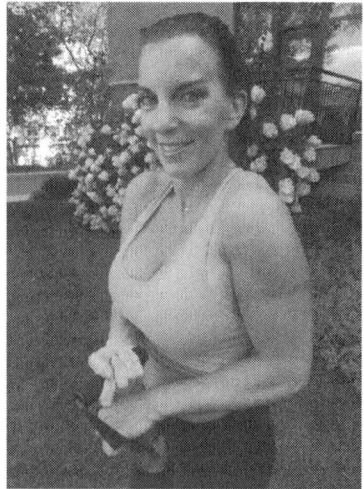

Breathe naturally and deeply in and out for about 10 full breaths, which will take about 1 second per breath. Aim to perform an exercise breathing count of no less than 7 seconds, and for no longer than 10 seconds.

Next, you'll need to perform the same exercise in reverse so that you now engage the biceps of your left arm, and triceps muscles of your right arm.

Iso-Bow® Biceps and Triceps Cradle Press-Curl (Right Side)

Cradle the Iso-Bow® with your right hand, gripping the top with your left hand facing up. Grip the cradled side of the Iso-Bow® with the right hand facing down.

Keep both elbows close to your body, and with your left arm across the front of you at waist height. In this position, press down with the right hand, and at the same time press up with the left, to engage both the Biceps and Triceps muscles simultaneously.

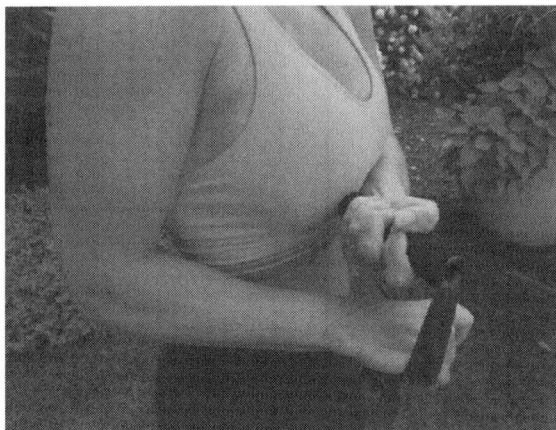

Breathe naturally and deeply in and out for about 10 full breaths, which will take about 1 second per breath.

Aim to perform an exercise breathing count of no less than 7 seconds, and for no longer than 10 seconds

Forearms

Iso-Bow® Seated Wrist Curl and Extension

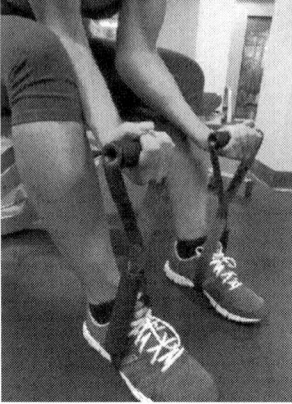

Place an Iso-Bow® around each foot, and hold both handles with your palms facing up, attempt to curl both wrists upwards, to engage the forearm muscles.

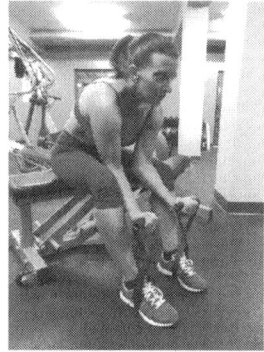

Breathe naturally and deeply in and out for about 10 full breaths, which

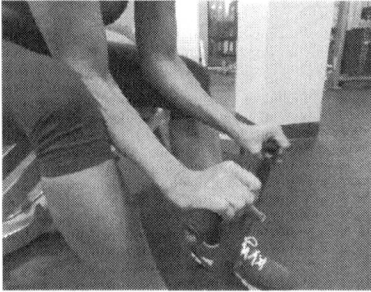

will take about 1 second per breath.

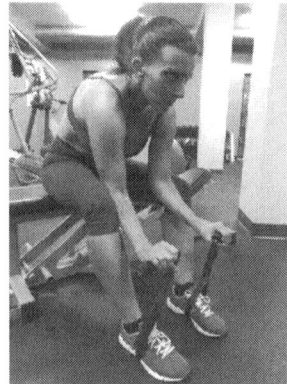

Aim to perform an exercise breathing count of no less than 7 seconds, and for no longer than 10 seconds. Switch your grip so that your palms are facing down, and repeat the exercise.

Lower Back

Dual Iso-Bow® Bent Leg Deadlift

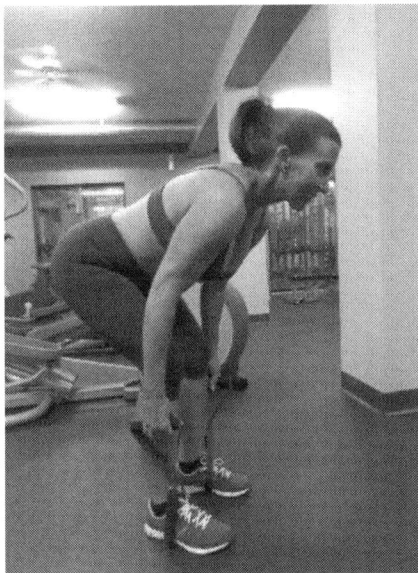

Place the loop handle of both Iso-Bows® around each foot as shown. Hold each handle firmly while maintaining a perfect bent-knee, semi squat position with your back straight at all times, then attempt to slowly stand up straight.

Engage the muscles of the glutes, hamstrings, lower back, thighs, and other core muscles,

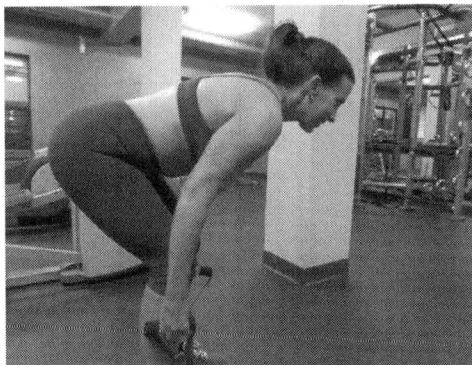

while the Iso-Bows® secured by your feet prevent any movement from taking place.

Breathe naturally and deeply in and out for about 10 full breaths, which will take about 1 second per breath.

Aim to perform an exercise breathing count of no less than 7 seconds, and for no longer than 10 seconds.

Abdominals

Iso-Bow® V-Sit Side to Side

Lay down, and raise your legs and torso off the floor by curling the spine, gripping the Iso-Bow® securely with both hands close to your mid-section.

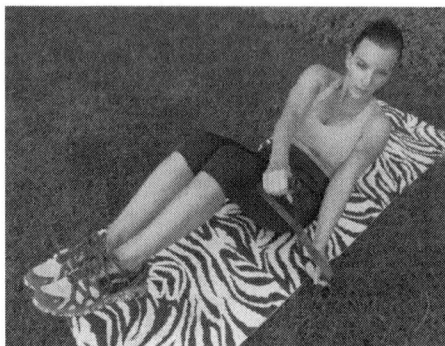

Twist the Iso-Bow® to one side as you engage the abdominal and oblique muscles.

Breathe naturally and deeply in and out for about 10 full breaths, which will take about 1 second per breath.

Aim to perform an exercise breathing count of no less than 7 seconds, and for no longer than 10 seconds. Repeat the exercise on the other side of your body.

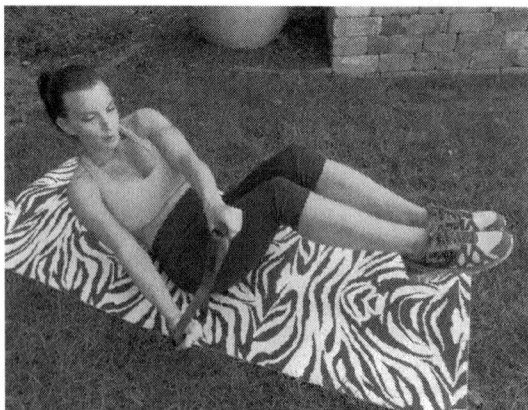

The ISO90™ Course Week 12 at a Glance

Legs – Upper Thighs

- ⚠ *Dual Iso-Bow® Stirrup Squat*
- ⚠ *Standing Hamstring Wall Curl – Left and Right Leg*

Calf's

- ⚠ *Calf Single Leg Wall Push – Left and Right Leg*

Upper Back

- ⚠ *Iso-Bow® Doorway Pull Ups*

Upper Back - Alternative to Pull Ups

- ⚠ *Dual Iso-Bow® Seated Foot-Stirrup Row*

Chest

- ⚠ *Iso-Bow® Chest Press and Upper Back Row – Left and Right*

Shoulders

- ⚠ *Iso-Bow® Single Arm Overhead Press – Left and Right Arm*
- ⚠ *Iso-Bow® Mid Hold Lateral Pull Apart - AKA Lateral Raise*

Arms

- ⚠ *Iso-Bow® Biceps and Triceps Cradle Press-Curl (Left Side)*
- ⚠ *Iso-Bow® Biceps and Triceps Cradle Press-Curl (Right Side)*

Forearms

- ⚠ *Iso-Bow® Seated Wrist Curl and Extension*

Lower Back

- ⚠ *Dual Iso-Bow® Bent Leg Deadlift*

Abdominals

- ⚠ *Iso-Bow® V-Sit Side to Side*

Conclusion

When you first read this section concluding The ISO90™ Course, it's almost certainly because you're skipping through various sections before you perform the course. However, when you eventually read this section as a natural progression, because you've completed the entire ISO90™ course, you'll now be stronger, fitter, and healthier. You'll also have made excellent progress in forging your body into the new size and shape you desire. In addition, many people will have made a great start on another journey, one which will completely overhaul their lifestyle and body shape for the long-term. Some people may even have already succeeded in creating the new body size, the strength, and body shape they've always wanted.

At this point, it's worth remembering that you've just completed a very demanding exercise course. One which was designed to gradually increase in intensity as the weeks progressed. Now you've reached week 12, it's probably a good idea to take short break from training, to allow your body to refresh itself from the demands that were placed upon it during the intense 90-day course.

We suggest that you take a rest period of one week, or more if required, from all training before you start exercising again. If you wish, for a few weeks you can perform the basic, but highly effective, advanced routine in "The 70 Second Difference™" book. This carefully planned 7-exercise course is deceptively powerful, and it exercises all the major muscle groups of the body. This powerful routine will help to ensure that you stay in great shape, and maintain your hard-won gains of strength, muscle, and body shape. Since the advanced 70 Second Difference™ routine only takes 70 seconds of consecutive exercise time to perform, it fit into any lifestyle, no matter how busy you are. When you're eventually ready to start another new, and more advanced routine again, you may even wish to put your own routine together by mixing up various exercises from different weeks in The ISO90™ Course to create your own progressive workout plan. The choice is yours, and there's plenty to choose from.

We'd like to sincerely thank you for performing The ISO90™ Course. We'd also like to encourage you to make an ISOfitness™ workout an integral part of your daily life. Helen Renée and I keep a pair of Iso-Bow® devices with us literally everywhere we go. More importantly, even while travelling in cars, on trains, on ships, and on planes, we always use them regularly to perform an intense, high-level exercise routine. You can do the same.

If you want more suggestions and ideas about new exercises you can perform, then you can always log onto the members side of the ISOfitness™ website. You'll find dozens of more isometric exercises and exercise variations, together with a growing number of other types of exercises. There will always be something new for you to try, or you may even find an old exercise that you like, but have simply forgotten about. Exercise boredom is NOT an option with the ISOfitness™ exercise system. Our already large exercise database is growing, as we continue to add new videos of new exercises. These will keep your exercise sessions varied, interesting, and exciting, it will help to ensure your continued success in fitness, body shaping and strength!

www.ISOfitness.us www.MajorVision.com www.ISOfitness.uk

The 70 Second Difference™

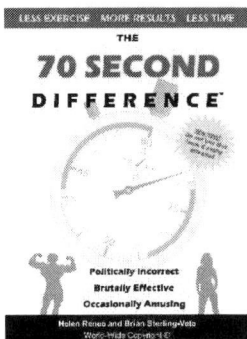

Stop confusing activity with accomplishment by exercising the traditional way with long exercise sessions, and with less than scientific guesses about how much and how many you need to do, of sets and repetitions.

Your time is too precious to waste, and time is the number 1 reason why people either stop exercising regularly, or don't exercise to begin with.

Big fitness club chains and gyms, want to make you believe that it takes hours of time each week, and that all their expensive and bulky equipment is essential for you to get a complete workout. You don't need all of this, and you certainly don't need to spend hours and hours of time each week just to exercise.

Just 70 seconds of focussed ISOfitness™ exercise daily has been scientifically proven to make you stronger, fitter, more muscular, and reduce your body fat. It will give you more results, with less exercise, and in less time than any other system because it's the appliance of science, NOT guesswork.

To many, The 70 Second Difference™ approach is controversial. However, this is almost certainly because we're openly focused only on proven science-based results, science-based exercise, and scientific data about nutrition. We also explain the science and the inconvenient truths

242

about many popular food sources, why bodybuilders and strength athletes are so physically different, how much protein you really need, weight control and weight loss, as well as the real science behind muscle growth and strength.

The 70 Second Difference™ approach to exercise utilises special short burst, highly focussed isometric exercises which are proven to be superior to old fashioned traditional exercise methods in over 5,500 independent scientific studies.

The 70 Second Difference™ explains how ISOfitness™ exercise engages your natural Adaptive Response™ mechanism, which means that everyone benefits from the same exercises in roughly equal percentages of improvement. This means that both unfit beginners and top professional athletes will all get the perfect workout that's right for them at their individual level of strength and fitness.

The 70 Second Difference™ is also a special workout routine using ISOfitness™ exercises. It is designed to give you a highly effective full-body workout in only 70 seconds of continuous exercise time.

Required Equipment: 2 x Iso-Bows® - available on Amazon.com, or direct from Bullworker.com

The Bullworker Bible™

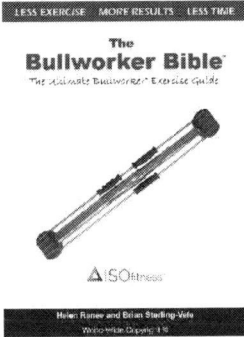

The Bullworker Bible™ is the definitive resource guide for all Bullworker® users, and it's the companion book for The Bullworker 90™ Course.

The Bullworker Bible™ is approved by the makers, and distributors of The Bullworker, at Bullworker.com

The Bullworker Bible™ is the complete science-based user-friendly guide of how the Bullworker should be used properly to deliver maximum results. It also shows you how to effectively use the Bow Extension® and the Steel Bow®.

It gives you all the information that you always wanted to know, but the simple wall charts, and very basic instruction manuals didn't.

- △ How Repetition-Compression Speed Control is Essential
- △ Correct Breathing Techniques
- △ Hooke's Law of Physics and The Bullworker™
- △ Correct Biomechanics for Best Results

The Bullworker Bible™ is also the essential guide for all users of the Bullworker X5, Bully Extreme, ISO 7x, and the Bullworker X7.

Brian Sterling-Vete is an internationally acclaimed exercise scientist and martial arts lifetime achievement award-winner who is also a 45+ year Bullworker® user. He used the Bullworker® to coach his friend and 4 times World's Strongest Man, Jon Pall Sigmarsson of Iceland.

Required Equipment: A Bullworker® Classic, or a similar device.

Recommended Additional Equipment: Steel Bow®, Bow Extension® kit, 2 x Iso-Bows®.

The Bullworker 90™ Course

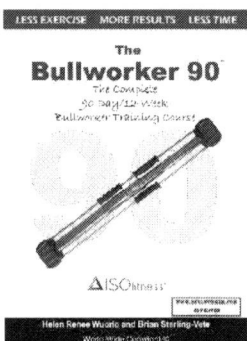

The Bullworker 90™ Course is the essential 90-day/12-week course for all Bullworker® users, and it's the companion book to The Bullworker Bible™

The Bullworker 90™ Course is approved by the makers, and distributors of The Bullworker, at Bullworker.com

The Bullworker 90™ is a 400+ page, science-based, user-friendly, step-by-step course designed to increase strength, fitness, grow muscle, body-build, and increase power over a 90-day/12-week period.

The Bullworker 90™ Course is a detailed exercise plan which progressively increases in intensity, as the days and weeks progress. New exercises are added almost every week, with complete routine changes every two weeks.

Each week has a detailed note section, together with suggestions about exercise days, and rest times etc., so that you know exactly what to do, and when to do it.

△ Step-by-step, week-by-week instruction

▲ Progressively increasing intensity over 90 days

▲ Routine changes every two weeks

▲ Isotonic and Isometric exercise combinations

▲ Multi-angle isometric exercise combinations

The Bullworker 90™ Course is designed by the authors of The Bullworker Bible™, and can be used with the Bullworker® Classic, the Steel Bow®, the Bullworker X5, the Bully Extreme, the ISO 7x, and the Bullworker X7.

The Bullworker 90™ Course also contains alternative/extra exercises which incorporate the use of the Iso-Bow®, and the Bow Extension®, that can be used with all Bullworker-type exercisers to increase the range and effectiveness of the device.

Required Equipment: A Bullworker® Classic, or a similar device.

Recommended Additional Equipment: Steel Bow®, Bow Extension® kit, 2 x Iso-Bows®.

Workout at Work™

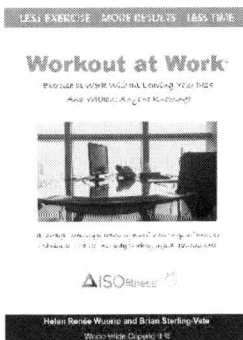

A stark new warning from the Icahn School of Medicine at Mount Sinai School of Medicine in New York reveals that sitting at a desk working for more than 6 hours a day can be extremely damaging to your health, and even exercising 4 evenings a week after work, or for long periods over the weekend, won't fix the damage.

The average person spends over 10 years of their life at work over an average 45 year working life, which for most people means sitting at a desk for a staggering 10-years of their life! Time, or lack of it, is also working against after-work exercise sessions. Exercising the traditional way in a gym 3-days a week, will consume a further 4.27 years. This is why time is the #1 reason why people don't exercise.

The fact is that sitting at a desk for more than 6 hours a day can cause potentially irreversible damage can be done to your heart, together with increases in both cholesterol and body fat, as well as insulin resistance which is a precursor to type 2 diabetes.

What if you could workout effectively while you were at work? What if a complete beginner could exercise with equal ease to someone who is an advanced athlete, and all without leaving your place of work?

Now you can do exactly that with The ISOfitness™ system of advanced isometric exercises. With the ISOfitness™ system, and a pair of Iso-Bows®, the world's smallest total-body exerciser, you can workout effectively at work, no matter what fitness level you're at, without ever leaving your desk!

Even if you perform just one 7-second high-intensity exercise every 30 minutes, you'll gain maximum benefit from this scientifically proven system. At the end of a 9-hour working day you can easily perform an 18-20 exercise total-body workout, so you leave work healthier, fitter, stronger, and with more time to spend with family and friends.

Your boss won't complain either, because in exchange for just 126 seconds out of your working day, you'll be up to 30% more efficient at your job, and you'll take less time off sick.

Required Equipment: 2 x Iso-Bows - available on Amazon.com

Fitness on the Move™

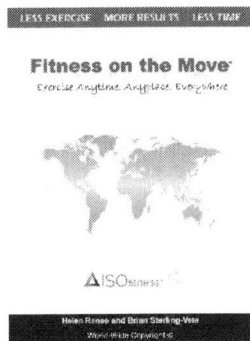

Time is the #1 reason why people don't exercise. The #2 reason is lack of access to a gym.

With the ISOfitness™ system of Fitness on the Move™ There are no more excuses. You can literally workout anytime, anyplace, everywhere, thanks to the ISOfitness™ exercise system of advanced isomeric exercises, combined with the powerful Iso-Bow®.

The advanced isometric exercises of the ISOfitness™ system have been scientifically proven in thousands of independent experiments to be superior to traditional exercise methods.

We've tried and tested the Fitness on the Move™ system by performing full workout routines as passengers in cars, on trains, in cramped airline seats, on mountainsides, on beaches, and once even on the deck of a ship in a storm.

The ISOfitness™ system of Fitness on the Move™ allows a full-body workout in the smallest space humanly possible thanks to our Zero Footprint Workout™ concept. With the Fitness on the Move™ system you never need to miss a workout ever again.

Required Equipment: 2 x Iso-Bows - available on Amazon.com, or direct from Bullworker.com

The SSASS™ Course

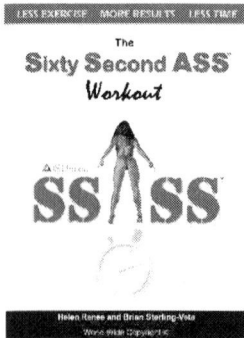

The Sixty Second ASS Workout™, or SSASS™ workout, is the fastest and most effective ass workout ever devised.

Based on the scientifically proven principles of the ISOfitness™ exercise system, the SSASS™ workout is a no-nonsense, no time-wasting workout that really does do everything you need to make your ass, tight, firm, shapely, and strong.

TIME, and more precisely the lack of it, is the #1 reason why people either don't exercise, or stop exercising. Life and work can just get in the way of exercise plans, and before you know it, it's been weeks since you had a workout.

The SSASS™ routine means no more time-wasting workouts where you twist, shake, waggle your ass, kick your legs, or dance around for 30 minutes. None of which really target the area you want. Time is short, and it's your choice if you want to waste it by waggling your ass to music because it "feels" good, or, if you want to get the job done in just 60 seconds of laser-focussed ISOfitness™ exercise.

Everyone has 60 seconds of time to spare, even on the busiest day, so, you're Just 60 seconds a day from having a great ass.

Required Equipment: 2 x Iso-Bows - available on Amazon.com, or direct from Bullworker.com

Mental Martial Arts

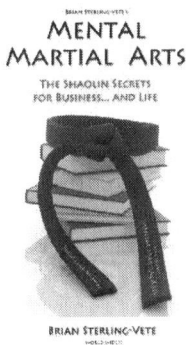

MENTAL
MARTIAL ARTS

THE SHAOLIN SECRETS
FOR BUSINESS... AND LIFE

BRIAN STERLING-VETE

Brian Sterling-Vete's Mental Martial Arts is a system of intellectual life-combat skills which uses the tactics and principles of the physical martial arts. All interaction in life, at your place of work, in your business, and when negotiating and communicating with others, is an exchange of energy, power and influence. During these interactions, one party is always exerting maximum influence over the other as they attempt to gain the outcome they prefer over the weaker party. The more powerful and persuasive will usually end as the winner. A physical analogy would be that of a bigger, stronger, and more powerful person gaining influence over a smaller, weaker person by bullying, intimidating, and even by physical violence. This is unless the apparently "weaker" person is trained in the martial arts...

Using Brian's unique system of Mental Martial Arts, you can learn to verbally, intellectually, and emotionally guide, channel, and redirect the energy of others, even more powerful people and large organisations. In doing so, you achieve the outcome you desire in both life and business. Brian's Mental Martial Arts system contains a specific section to help those who may be forced to face a potentially hostile media in the event of a crisis. In this section, Brian combines his system of Mental Martial Arts, together with the experience he gained in over a decade with BBC TV News, to help you and your organisation stay "Media Safe." www.mentalmartialarts.tv

Tuxedo Warriors

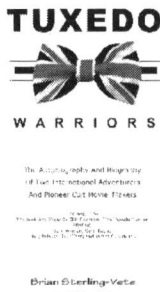

Tuxedo Warriors is the companion book to The Tuxedo Warrior. This is the autobiography of author, composer, movie-maker Cliff Twemlow. The book ended at the beginning of what has been called the Golden Age of Video Cinematography, which he inspired.

The new book, Tuxedo Warriors is the most complete biography of Cliff Twemlow ever written. It's also the autobiography Brian Sterling-Vete, who played a central role in this unique, entertaining, and true story of two extraordinary "Renaissance-Men," and their adventures as guerrilla movie-makers.

Brian and Cliff traversed the globe on many previously untold adventures in Iceland, and the Arctic Circle, in the Mediterranean, in North Africa and a war zone, on tramp-steamer journeys across the ocean, and on road trips across continents.

Tuxedo Warriors is told by Brian Sterling-Vete, and he continues the story where the original book ends. Brian is perhaps the only person who can tell the complete story from the time it all began, right through until the end, with sudden and untimely death of his great friend Cliff.

Cliff and his works have now become known globally, even achieving "cult" status, primarily thanks to great work of Dr Chris Lee and Andy Wills in their excellent book "The Lost World of CLIFF TWEMLOW: The King of Manchester Exploitation Movies," re-releases of his movies, and through TV documentaries.

Tuxedo Warriors is a compelling, entertaining, and true story about two extraordinary characters who were pioneers during this pivotal and innovative period in the history of world cinema. Tuxedo Warriors is the sequel to the book, and movie by Cliff Twemlow: "The Tuxedo Warrior," Starring: John Wyman, Carol Royle, Holly Palance, John Terry and James Coburn Jnr.

The Tuxedo Warrior by Cliff Twemlow – Prologue and epilogue by Brian Sterling-Vete

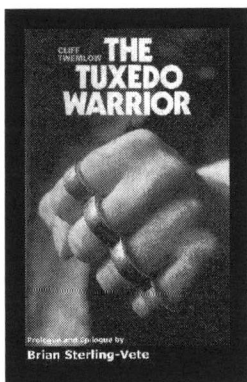

There are many ways in which a Doorman can gain respect. Numerous methods applied to the principal. In my profession, every available technique must be utilised, depending on the situation and circumstances.

Would-be transgressors either move-off the premises quietly acknowledging your diplomatic approach. Or, the other alternative whereby physical persuasion has to be exercised, which either quells their pugilistic desires, or it triggers their aggressive instincts, turning the whole incident into a bloody and violent encounter.

'The Tuxedo Warrior,' pulls no punches in its brawling, savage, colourful, and entertaining exposure of society's nightlife activities.

The above, is the original text from the rear cover of Cliff's book. Cliff and I were extremly close friends, and I'm honoured to re-publish his original work, which completes the storyline of my own book, 'Tuxedo Warriors.'

Where Cliff's original book ends, my own book overlaps and begins, to complete his colourful life story. I'm also honoured to be close friends with his eldest son, Barry Twemlow, and sincerely thank him for writing a foreword to make this re-published book all the more complete.

The Pike by Cliff Twemlow – Prologue and epilogue by Brian Sterling-Vete

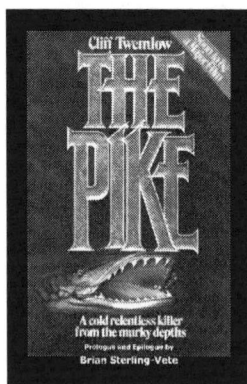

ITS FIRST VICTIMS

A screeching swan… A fisherman overboard… A drunken woman…

One by one, the mysterious killer in Lake Windermere claims its terrified victims. Tearing off limbs with its monstrous teeth, horribly mutilating bodies.

Fear sweeps the peaceful holiday resort when experts identify the creature as a giant pike…. A hellish creature with the strength to rupture boats, and the anger to attack them.

But for some, the terror becomes a bonanza—the traders who cater to the gathering crowds of ghouls on the shore. And, they will do anything to stop divers finding the creature. Meanwhile the ripples of bloodshed widen....
The Pike

The above, is the original text from the rear cover of Cliff's book. I remember this book going into pre-production as a major movie in the early 1980's starring Joan Collins. Sadly, the financiers ran into personal difficulties and it was never made.

Today, there is now renewed interest in this book as a screenplay and movie. In my own book, 'Tuxedo Warriors,' I tell the behind the scenes story of myself, my close friend Cliff Twemlow, and The Pike.

The Beast of Kane by Cliff Twemlow – Prologue and epilogue by Brian Sterling-Vete

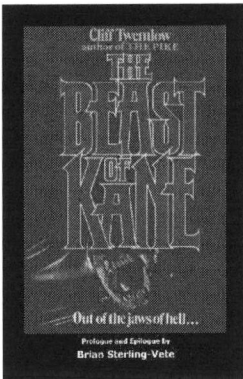

When the Gordon Family open their door to a stray Elkhound, they unwittingly welcome-in the forces of evil. For, according to the local priest, the huge dog is Satan himself, fulfilling an ancient prophecy.

But, no one will believe this warning... Even when sheep – and wolves – are mysteriously slaughtered. Even when frenzied pets turn on their owners. Even when Emily Forrest is savagely eaten alive – the first of many human victims. As winter tightens its icy grip on the remote town of Kane, its unprotected people must face an unearthly terror.

The above, is the original text from the rear cover of Cliff's book.   This was the first of Cliff's books to be accepted by Hammer Film Studios to be made into a big-screen horror movie, along with Cliff's other book, The Pike.

More importantly, the reason why it was never to be made into a movie was no reflection on the book itself. It was entirely because of the increasing financial challenges Hammer Films were facing at that time.   They were issues that were so serious, that they caused the unexpected and rapid decline of the studio.

www.ISOfitness.us www.majorvision.com www.ISOfitness.uk

Printed in Great Britain
by Amazon